MICRODOSING

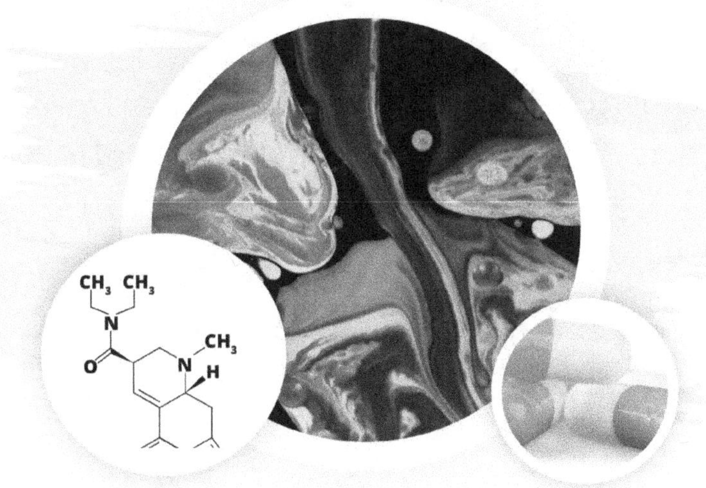

MACROBENEFITS IN HEALTH AND WELL-BEING. YOUR BODY IN PSYCHEDELIC AND NON-PSYCHEDELIC SUBSTANCES

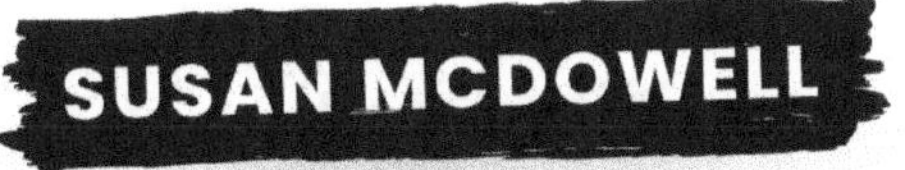

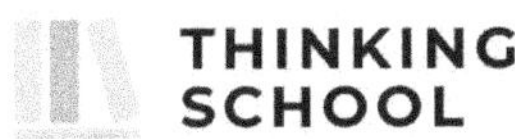

MICRODOSING

Macrobenefits in health and well-being. Your body in psychedelic and non-psychedelic substances

- Susan McDowell -

Microdosing / Susan McDowell – 1st Edition

ISBN 9798321396209

INDEX

PREAMBLE OF A FIELD TO BE EXPLORED

In recent years, clinical studies and laboratory research have revealed that psychedelics, when administered in a supportive, controlled setting, can improve mood disorders such as severe depression, anxiety, and posttraumatic stress disorder. Now, a growing number of scientists are exploring whether these potent substances could also be effective in treating physical injuries to the brain and other disorders resulting from an altered brain configuration. This could have significant implications for conditions such as strokes, traumatic brain injuries, Alzheimer's, and Parkinson's.

Psychedelics are a class of consciousness-altering compounds, including lysergic acid diethylamide (LSD), psilocybin (present in magic mushrooms), methylenedioxymethamphetamine (MDMA or ecstasy), dimethyltryptamine (DMT), and ayahuasca (a drink derived from certain plants in South America), among others. Each of these compounds affects the brain slightly differently.

A pioneering imaging study in Biological Psychiatry: Cognitive Neuroscience and Neuroimaging sheds light on how the brain functions under the influence of psychedelic drugs and their potential for treating psychiatric disorders.

The study reveals that psilocybin, a compound found in "magic mushrooms," triggers a pattern of hyperconnectivity in the brain associated with ego-dissolving effects and feelings of oceanic boundlessness. Published by Elsevier, the findings help explain the mystical experiences reported during psychedelic use and are relevant for the therapeutic use of psychedelics in treating disorders such as depression.

Oceanic boundlessness encompasses a sense of unity, blissfulness, insightfulness, and spiritual experiences typically associated with psychedelic sessions.

In one of the first brain imaging studies of its kind, researchers discovered a specific link between the psychedelic state and dynamic changes in whole-brain connectivity. While previous research has shown increases in static global brain connectivity under psychedelics, this study demonstrates that hyperconnectivity is dynamic (changing over time) and that its transition rate correlates with feelings of oceanic boundlessness, a hallmark of the psychedelic state.

Lead investigator Johannes G. Ramaekers, PhD, from Maastricht University, states, "Psilocybin has been extensively studied for its potential to treat various disorders, including obsessive-compulsive disorder, death-related anxiety, depression, treatment-resistant depression, major depressive disorder, terminal cancer-associated anxiety, demoralization, and addictions to smoking and alcohol. However, the brain activity underlying these profound experiences was not fully understood."

Psilocybin induces significant changes at both the brain and experiential levels. The brain's tendency to enter a hyperconnected-hyperarousal state under psilocybin suggests the potential for experiencing different mental perspectives. This study illuminates the intricate relationship between brain dynamics and subjective experiences under psilocybin, providing insights into the neurophysiology and experiential qualities of the psychedelic state.

Dr. Ramaekers adds, "Our analyses suggest that psilocybin alters brain function, making the overall neurobiological pattern more connected, fluid, and less modular."

Using previously acquired functional magnetic resonance imaging (fMRI) data, the study analyzed two groups: one group of 22 individuals received a single dose of psilocybin, while the other 27 participants received a placebo. During the peak effects of the drug, participants who received psilocybin reported significant phenomenological changes compared to the placebo group. Brain connectivity analysis revealed a pattern of global region-to-region connectivity reappearing over time in the psilocybin group, potentially accounting for the varied mental associations participants experienced.

Moreover, this hyperconnected pattern was linked to oceanic boundlessness and unity, indicating an important mapping between brain dynamics and subjective experience. This suggests "egotropic effects" (ego-modifying) of the drug are significant compared to hallucinogenic effects.

Larry Fort, a PhD candidate and co-author from the University of Liège, emphasizes, "Psychedelic drugs like psilocybin are often referred to as hallucinogens. We expected hallucinatory experiences to correlate highest with psilocybin's hyperconnected pattern. However, ego-modifying experiences had a stronger correlation, leading us to introduce the term 'egotropic' to highlight these effects."

Cameron S. Carter, MD, Editor-in-Chief of Biological Psychiatry: Cognitive Neuroscience and Neuroimaging, comments, "This study uses readily available resting-state fMRI images after psilocybin ingestion to provide new insights into the neurophysiological mechanisms underlying the drug's subjective and clinical effects. It paves the way for future studies using other psychedelic agents to explore whether these dynamic connectivity effects are a general mechanism for the therapeutic benefits of these compounds."

Athena Demertzi, PhD, from the University of Liège, adds, "We were pleasantly surprised to find that the hyperconnected brain pattern was also characterized by lower global signal amplitude, a proxy for heightened cortical arousal. This is the first time such an approximation has been attempted in psychedelic research, and it may be important as we move towards fully characterizing brain states under psychedelics."

She concludes, "With the resurgence of research into the psychotherapeutic applications of psychedelics, our results are crucial for understanding how subjective experiences under psychedelics lead to beneficial clinical outcomes. Is the effect driven by ego-dissolution or hallucinations? Our work shows how the strong relationship between the egotropic effects of moderate dose psilocybin and its hyperconnected brain pattern can guide clinical focus on specific aspects of phenomenology, such as ego-dissolutions. This information can help healthcare professionals design psychedelic therapy sessions to achieve the best clinical outcomes."

So far, most brain injury research, conducted in test tubes and laboratory animals with only a few human studies, suggests the potential of psychedelics to limit post-injury brain damage, stimulate neurogenesis to replace damaged neurons, and reopen learning windows that enable the brain to acquire new skills. A recent study revealed that laboratory animals treated with psychedelics developed skills in adulthood that were normally limited to childhood.

These drugs may be especially valuable because brain lesions often lack effective therapies.

Human brains develop so that certain skills are easier to learn during specific critical periods. A commonly understood analogy is learning a new language in adulthood, as the critical period for language usually closes after adolescence.

However, scientists at Johns Hopkins University in the United States reported that adult rodents given a psychedelic drug learned social skills that are typically acquired only in their youth.

This finding has implications for the treatment of strokes and traumatic brain injuries (TBIs). When someone experiences these injuries, many brain cells are damaged. Fortunately, a critical period for speech learning and motor skills naturally reopens after the event, allowing the person to regain some lost skills. However, it usually closes within six months, making it difficult to improve after that time.

In the study, adult mice lacking certain social skills were trained to associate a specific environment with loneliness and another with social interaction. After receiving a single dose of LSD, psilocybin, or another psychedelic, mice could choose to spend time in either setting. Most preferred the social environment.

All psychedelics produced this effect, but those that caused longer psychedelic experiences in humans reopened the critical mouse period for longer afterwards. For example, with LSD, whose effects last about 10 hours, mice continued to learn about the importance of socialization for months afterward, compared to weeks for psychedelics with shorter hallucinations.

This is likely because psychedelics such as LSD remain at receptors for a long time, overloading neurons and triggering a kind of reset, similar to a full restart after a computer crashes. This cascade of cellular events restarts the brain to an earlier stage of development.

Reopening the learning windows explains why psychedelic studies for mood disorders emphasize the importance of post-drug psychotherapy, known as integration. During integration, the brain is open to new ideas, allowing it to address mental illness in innovative ways.

Reopening the learning windows can also be beneficial for people whose brains are connected differently, such as those with autism spectrum disorder (ASD), a neurologic and developmental disorder that affects, among other things, how they interact socially. Research has shown that the brains of people with autism have some differences, especially in the frontal cortex, which regulates emotions and relationships, compared with those without autism.

In a study conducted at the University of California, USA, eight adults with autism spectrum disorder experienced a marked reduction in social anxiety after receiving two doses of MDMA, each followed by three sessions of psychotherapy. The benefits of this therapy persisted through the six months of follow-up.

MDMA could be especially valuable for autism because it facilitates the desire to socialize, a skill that many on the spectrum find challenging. Under the effects of MOTAPM, one experiences a deep desire to interact with others in a non-aggressive, pro-social and empathetic way.

Other ways psychedelics seem to influence the brain include reducing inflammation, a major contributor to damage after brain injury. Although inflammation is a useful biological response to injured tissue because it attracts immune cells and other healing chemicals, too much of it can be problematic.

Several labs are investigating the psychedelic DMT as a possible treatment to boost recovery after a stroke. DMT works by stimulating another type of receptor called sigma-1 (S1R), which seems to play a crucial role in protecting cells against damage that occurs when blood flows to the brain after a stroke.

Experiments in rats given low doses of DMT after a stroke showed less damaged tissue and more complete recovery; in addition, brain levels of anti-inflammatory compounds and sigma-1 proteins were higher in treated animals.

Traumatic brain injuries, which result from violent head impacts such as car crashes or explosions, are especially challenging to treat because of their ability to damage multiple areas of the brain.

It has been suggested that new psychedelics designed to prevent altered consciousness could be especially effective in treating brain injuries. This idea has been strengthened by recent research finding that, in addition to binding to serotonin 5-HT2A receptors, psychedelics also attach to a receptor called TrkB, which facilitates communication between nerve cells. Although antidepressants also activate this receptor, psychedelics are much more potent.

TrkB has no hallucinogenic effects, suggesting that drugs designed to target these receptors without activating 5HT2A may provide similar curative benefits. Unlike mood disorders, where some consider the psychedelic appearance to be important for treatment, it may be less crucial for brain injuries.

Many clinicians and researchers point out that the advantage of psychedelic therapies lies in their potency, which usually means that only one or a few doses are needed. This offers a unique treatment pathway compared with many current drugs for brain injuries, which often require daily doses.

On the vast horizon of medical knowledge and the pursuit of human well-being, there is a path less explored but full of promise and potential. This book is an invitation to enter that fascinating and often misunderstood path, where microdoses of natural substances and innovative compounds offer a window into a world of possibilities for improving our mental, emotional, and physical health.

For decades, traditional medical practices have been the foundation of health care, but as science and technology advance, new ways of understanding and addressing health and well-being also emerge. In this context, microdoses rise as an exciting prospect, a convergence between ancient wisdom and modern research.

Substances now widely classified as psychedelic have a long history of healthy use among the Indigenous peoples of the Americas/Turtle Island, including the Mazatec, Huichol, Shipibo and other nations, as well as the pre-Columbian Mayan, Olmec, Zapotec and Aztec societies.

These indigenous health technologies have been subject to centuries of repression, first through colonization and the Inquisition of the Americas, and then by the US-led "war on drugs." However, they have re-emerged in recent decades as drugs with the potential to address mental illness and improve well-being among largely non-Indigenous communities.

Although this interest has focused predominantly on sufficient doses to generate dramatic alterations in consciousness, the use of smaller microdoses, absent of the profound sensory and cognitive effects that typify the psychedelic experience, is also a subject of substantial interest in psychedelic interest groups, popular culture, and emerging scientific literature.

Over time, there arises a moment when the confines of physical limitations begin to blur as the power of your mind surges forth. In this transformative juncture, you find yourself venturing into realms previously deemed unreachable, guided by the intrepid spirit of exploration. What once seemed beyond the scope of possibility now beckons invitingly, urging you to traverse landscapes of thought and experience hitherto uncharted.

This journey of mental liberation is a testament to the remarkable capacity of the human psyche to transcend its own confines. It represents a convergence of inner resilience and external stimuli, propelling you towards the realization of aspirations once deemed unattainable. As your mind stretches its wings, you discover newfound depths of courage and imagination, embarking on a voyage of self-discovery and boundless potential.

In fact, while long-term consumption of higher doses of psilocybin-containing mushrooms is well documented among Mazatecans in Mexico, the use of smaller microdoses to support healing of physical conditions and emotional states such as sadness, anger, envy, isolation, and agitation is also common among Mazatecans.

The exact parameters of what constitutes a microdose and the associated practice of regular microdosing have not yet been firmly articulated; however, it has been generally described that microdosing involves successive self-administration within a limited period of time of doses of psychedelic drugs that do not affect normal functioning and are predominantly subsensory[8]. Psilocybin and LSD are substances used by the vast majority of participants in observational and retrospective microdosing research.

The reported microdoses identified in the observational investigation usually range from 5 to 20 µg LSD and from 0.1 to 0.3 g of dried psilocybin mushrooms. Microdoses are most used several times a week in various alternate day patterns9,10. The single study comparing the frequency of microdosing between DNC and psilocybin users reported equivalent patterns of use between substances but did not examine differences in relative dose.

In addition to the microdosing of psychedelics alone, the growing interest has focused on a practice known colloquially as stacking that involves combining microdoses of psychedelics—mainly mushrooms containing psilocybin—with other substances proposed to accentuate the health effects.

The use of such mixtures appears to have a long history; Aztecs combined cocoa with psilocybin mushrooms in a practice known as "cacahua-xochitl", which literally means "chocolate mushrooms"18, and psilocybin mixtures composed of honey, flowers and herbs have been noted in historical records among both Indigenous and non-Indigenous peoples.

Following a similar profile, mushrooms, henbane (also known as night umbrella, Hyoscyamus niger), stinging nettles (Urtica dioica) and other active substances were commonly added to increase the effects of beer during the Middle Ages until the approval, in 1516, of the German Reinheitsgebot, also known as the Bavarian Purity Law. Chocolate and cocoa remain popular additions to psilocybin, while the addition of Syrian rue (Peganum harmala), lion mane mushrooms (Hericium erinaceus) and/or niacin appear to be more recent phenomena.

Similar to the practice of microdosing more generally, the popularity of stacking probably stems from the proliferation of positive anecdotal reports over the past decade rather than from a solid empirical basis. In fact, as far as we know, no studies have been conducted that have directly tested the possible synergistic effects of these substances when combined with psilocybin. Therefore, the proposed mechanisms of action, benefits, and subjective effects of psilocybin stacked microdose mixtures are usually derived from reports associated with the substance stacked alone.

Unlike a drug addict who loses their resourcefulness over time, the lessons you gain from navigating high-risk situations remain with you long after the immediate intensity has faded. Engaging in risky endeavors sharpens your focus and heightens your senses, forcing you to develop quick thinking and adaptive strategies. These experiences carve out a set of skills and insights that become a permanent part of your cognitive toolkit. While the acute sharpness you once felt in the heat of the moment may dull, the knowledge and abilities you acquired endure, forming a resilient foundation for future challenges. Either way, this book is not about risks, but containment. It is about microdosing.

The value of what you have learned under pressure transcends the transient nature of the risk itself. This hard-earned wisdom cannot be easily taken from you, unlike the fleeting euphoria of substance abuse that erodes personal capabilities over time. The growth derived from high-risk experiences fortifies your mental resilience and problem-solving acumen. Consequently, even as the vividness of those moments diminishes, the core competencies and confidence gained remain, empowering you to tackle new obstacles with a deeper understanding and a well-honed skill set.

For example, the benefits of cocoa and the potential cognitive-enhancing properties of Lion's Mane mushrooms have been proposed to create synergies with the supposedly complementary qualities of psilocybin mushrooms. Other reasons for stacking include observations about possible biochemical interactions. Specifically, both Syrian Rue and Lion's Mane have been identified as monoamine oxidase inhibitors (MAOIs), and MAOIs have a long history of use in psychedelic mixtures such as ayahuasca, where they serve to extend and enhance the effects of 5HT2a receptor agonists.

In contrast, the washout effects of niacin are suggested to facilitate psilocybin bioavailability and be prophylactic for abuse. However, despite traditional practices, theoretical justification, and contemporary anecdote suggesting the potential benefits of stacking, empirical studies of most stacked substances are limited and largely involve animal models.

Therefore, caution should be exercised when interpreting claims related to the synergistic effects of stacked substances and psilocybin in humans.

The practice of microdosing seems to have increased substantially in the last decade and recent studies have begun to characterize individuals who use microdoses. Comparisons with community samples that do not contain microdoses generally identify few differences between microdosers and non-microdosers. However, some findings suggest that, like psychedelic users more generally, microdosers are disproportionately male and lower in education and income compared to non-microdosers. Interestingly, microdosers report higher levels of substance use in the past year, but lower levels of substance use disorders, anxiety disorders and negative emotionality.

Surveys identify various motivations for microdosing; respondents point to reducing anxiety and depression, improving well-being, and increasing cognitive performance as key motivations; less prominent motivations include improving physical health and increasing empathy, spirituality, and curiosity.

The importance of addressing mental health problems and improving psychological well-being and cognition suggests that a substantial proportion of those who microdose may be doing so in an attempt to treat symptoms of mental illness or prevent cognitive decline. In fact, microdosers report reduced stress, improved mood, and attenuated symptoms of depression, anxiety, post-traumatic stress disorder, and obsessive-compulsive disorder. Studies have also reported that microdosing may be perceived as more effective than conventional treatments for psychiatric symptoms.

Findings from the prospective microdosing study alone suggest positive changes in most psychologic domains on microdose days relative to baseline days, and cross-sectional findings suggest lower levels of dysfunctional attitudes and negative emotionality and higher levels of positive mood. However, although one study has investigated the lifetime prevalence of psychiatric disorders among microdosers, no study has estimated the extent to which psychological differences between microdosers and non-microdosers vary according to history and mental health reasons.

My aim is to contribute to the microdosing literature by further characterizing microdosers and microdosing practices, including a detailed assessment of the combination of psychedelic and non-psychedelic substances (i.e., stacking).

We evaluated the differences between microdosers and controls on symptoms of depression, anxiety, and stress among participants with mental health problems and examined the relationships between motivation for microdosing and mental health. Finally, the consistency of microdosing practices and motivations across gender and mental health are investigated.

As we go into the following chapters, we will explore the non-psychedelic and psychedelic substances that have captured the attention of the medical and scientific community. We will investigate the scientific evidence and empirical experience that support its use in microdoses, and consider both its potential effects and its limitations. We will delve into philosophical and ethical debates, explore their integration into medical practice and envision the future of this exciting field.

Also, there is a limit and an elephant in the room that needs to be addressed. For someone caught in the throes of addiction, it is not merely the euphoric highs that hold them captive, but rather the stark, dizzying contrast between the lows and the highs. In this tumultuous cycle, each descent into the depths of despair amplifies the allure of the subsequent ascent to euphoria. The addict becomes ensnared not only by the fleeting moments of ecstasy but also by the relentless pursuit of escaping the crushing weight of their own despair.

This addiction to extremes creates a relentless rollercoaster of emotions, where the rush of elation serves as a fleeting reprieve from the agony of withdrawal and emptiness. The addict finds themselves perpetually chasing the elusive high, driven by an insatiable craving for that dizzying rush of sensation. Yet, in this relentless pursuit, they become trapped in a cycle of dependency, unable to break free from the relentless grip of their addiction.

Microdosing is not about the highs and lows but about a safe and consistent way to explore a new depth in our own psyche.

This book is not intended to be a definitive guide, but rather a beacon of light in a sea of possibilities. I invite you to join me in this journey, opening your mind to the new and challenging perspectives that microdoses offer us. Through this journey of discovery and exploration, I hope you will find inspiration to make informed and courageous decisions in search of greater well-being and a deeper understanding of the wonder that is the human mind.

FUNDAMENTALS OF MICRODOSES

EXPLORING THE FOUNDATIONS OF AN ANCIENT AND CONTEMPORARY PRACTICE

The history of medicine is woven with threads of innovation, discovery, and sometimes even intrigue. In this chapter, we will take the first steps towards the vast world of microdoses, a practice that has been present throughout human history and that, in recent times, has resurfaced with renewed interest and potential.

At the heart of microdoses lies a fundamental question: how can tiny amounts of substances, often from natural sources, have a noticeable impact on human physiology and psychology? As we enter this territory of exploration, it will be essential to unravel the fundamental concepts that underpin this practice, understanding its historical evolution, its intersection with traditional and alternative medicine, and the scientific principles that support it.

Throughout this chapter, we will break down the concept of microdoses into its most basic elements. We will explore how these tiny, often barely perceptible doses can trigger chain reactions in the body and mind. At the same time, we will observe how this practice is integrated into the broader panorama of therapeutic approaches, highlighting its similarities and differences with traditional medicine.

Microdoses are not simply a modern notion; their history goes back to ancient civilizations that experimented with plants and substances to achieve specific effects. Throughout the following pages, we will travel back in time to discover the historical roots of microdoses and their role in the pursuit of well-being and the expansion of consciousness.

As we venture into this journey of discovery, it is important to keep the mind open and the spirit curious. Microdoses invite us to question our perceptions of medicine, to challenge established norms, and to explore new forms of healing and personal growth. Join me as we unravel the fundamentals of microdoses and step into a terrain where science, tradition and the avant-garde converge in search of greater understanding and wellbeing.

Welcome to this fascinating journey into the fundamentals of microdoses.

DEFINITION OF MICRODOSES AND THEIR HISTORICAL EVOLUTION

Microdosing is a therapeutic and self-exploration practice that involves ingesting or administering small amounts of psychoactive substances or natural compounds for the purpose of obtaining subtle benefits in the mind and body, without experiencing the full psychedelic effects associated with higher doses. Often, these doses are so small that they do not cause perceptible alterations in perception but instead focus on stimulating neurologic, hormonal, or emotional processes in a more subtle way.

The historical evolution of microdoses is woven into the rich fabric of human exploration of plants and natural compounds for therapeutic and spiritual purposes. Although the practice is now associated with the resurgence of alternative medicine and scientific research, its origin can be traced back to ancient civilizations and cultures that used small doses of plants and herbs in rituals and ceremonies.

In various Indigenous cultures, shamans and healers have used substances in low doses to obtain specific effects on the mind and body. These rituals were considered a form of communication with the spiritual world and focused on the search for knowledge, healing, and expansion of consciousness. This historical background reveals that the notion of using lesser amounts of substances for therapeutic purposes has deep roots in human history.

As societies evolved and advanced in their scientific understandings, many of these ancient practices were relegated or even banned because of ethical, religious, and political concerns. However, in the second half of the 20th century, with the rise of the psychedelic movement and the scientific exploration of substances such as LSD and psilocybin, microdoses began to capture the attention of scientists, doctors, and enthusiasts of self-exploration.

In the 1960s, the countercultural movement and the proliferation of psychedelic research influenced the popularization of microdoses. Advocates of such practices argued that subperceptual doses of psychedelic substances could have therapeutic and creative benefits without the overwhelming effects of higher doses.

But, as psychedelic drugs were stigmatized and banned in many parts of the world, interest in microdoses waned for a few decades. It was only in the last few years that microdoses re-emerged as a subject of public research and discussion. Growing evidence of potential benefits and interest in addressing mental health and wellness issues have reinvigorated interest in the practice.

Today, microdosing is at an inflection point. The combination of more rigorous scientific research, openness to unconventional therapeutic approaches, and a growing interest in mental health and integral wellbeing has led to a resurgence of practice in a variety of contexts. The historical evolution of microdoses demonstrates their ability to adapt and transform over time, reflecting the continuing human quest for healing and the deep understanding of the mind and body.

In contemporary times, the evolution of microdoses has been marked by a combination of scientific research, public interest, and changes in cultural perception. As some legal restrictions have been relaxed and discussion about mental health and wellbeing has broadened, microdoses have found more fertile ground for exploration and development.

The 2000s and early 2010s marked a shift in public perception of psychedelic substances. With a new generation of researchers interested in studying the therapeutic and neuronal effects of these substances, the focus on microdoses was renewed. Studies of psilocybin, LSD, and other substances began to show promising results in treating depression, anxiety, and posttraumatic stress disorder.

The popularization of microdoses has also been facilitated by social networks and easy access to information. Online platforms have allowed people to share their subjective experiences with microdoses, generating virtual communities of individuals who share similar interests and goals. This has contributed to the spread of knowledge about microdoses and has helped to bring down stigmas associated with their use.

As mental health approaches become more holistic and patient-centered, microdoses have gained traction as an additional tool in the therapeutic arsenal. However, its evolution has also been marked by challenges and controversies. Lack of regulation and limitations in research still raise questions about its long-term safety and efficacy.

The future of microdoses looks promising, but also uncertain. As research advances and society adapts to new health paradigms, microdoses are likely to continue to evolve in their therapeutic and cultural role. Proper integration into medical practice and broader therapeutic approaches will depend on collaboration among scientists, medical professionals, policymakers, and the wider community.

The story of microdoses is a story of resilience, adaptation, and continuous search. From the practices of ancient healers to innovative scientific research, these small doses have captured the imagination and interest of generations. As we look to the future, what was once considered a margin could very well become an integral part of the landscape of human health and well-being.

PSYCHEDELIC SUBSTANCES IN NATIVE AMERICAN CULTURE

The history of substance use in Native American culture is a fascinating account of the interaction between plants and humans in the search for spiritual connections, healing, and knowledge. For millennia, Native American tribes and communities have had a deep and respectful relationship with nature, using a variety of sacred and enteogenic plants for ceremonial and medicinal purposes.

From the peyote used by the native tribes of the southwestern United States to the ayahuasca used by Amazonian cultures, substances have played a significant role in rituals seeking connection with the spiritual world and understanding of nature and the cosmos. These ceremonies, often conducted under the guidance of shamans and spiritual leaders, are regarded as ways of communicating with the gods, ancestors, and spirits of nature.

Indigenous wisdom recognizes the importance of using these substances with respect and reverence. Entheogenic experiences were seen as a way to learn profound lessons and receive spiritual revelations, as well as to address physical and mental health issues. The focus was not only on the effects of the substances themselves, but also on the ritual context and sacred purpose behind their consumption.

As history progressed and interactions with European colonizers changed cultural dynamics, many of these traditional practices were banned and suppressed due to cultural misunderstandings and the imposition of Western values. However, the wisdom and knowledge of these traditions did not completely disappear, and in recent decades there has been a resurgence in interest and research on the use of substances in native cultures.

The different uses of substances in Native American culture represent a complex interaction between spirituality, traditional medicine, and the connection with nature. Across Native American tribes and communities, a variety of substances have been used for ritual, healing, and ceremonial purposes, reflecting these cultures' deep understanding of the relationship between humans and the natural world.

One of the best-known examples is the use of peyote by native tribes in the southwestern United States. Peyote, a cactus containing the psychoactive substance mescaline, has been considered sacred and used in religious ceremonies such as peyote rhythm, intended to establish a deep connection with the spiritual world and ancestors. For these communities, the peyote is a gateway to understanding transcendence and divinity, as well as being valued for its supposed healing benefits.

In Amazonian cultures, the use of ayahuasca has been a fundamental element in their shamanic practices. Ayahuasca, a combination of plants containing dimethyltryptamine (DMT) and a monoamine oxidase inhibitor (MAOI), is consumed in shaman-led ceremonies to induce altered states of consciousness that allow them to access spiritual visions and communicate with spirits. These experiences are considered as ways to obtain knowledge and guidance in community and personal decision-making.

Tobacco is another substance of importance in many Native American cultures. Used in purification rituals and as an offering to spirits, tobacco is considered a tool of communication between the spiritual and earthly worlds. Native Americans believe that tobacco smoke brings their prayers and desires to the gods and spirits, establishing a deep spiritual connection during ceremonies and moments of reflection.

It is essential to recognize that these uses of substances in Native American culture are not based on hedonism or the pursuit of psychoactive experience, but on the belief that plants have spiritual and medicinal properties that can be channeled for the benefit of the community and the individual. However, it is essential to address these issues with respect and cultural sensitivity, considering the traditions and values of these communities, as well as avoiding misappropriation.

Today, the relationship with these substances is a complex and sensitive issue. While some continue to practice these traditions in a respectful and culturally appropriate manner, others seek a balance between tradition and innovation, exploring how these substances could be used to improve mental health, healing, and wellbeing in the context of contemporary medicine.

The history of substance use in Native American culture is a testament to the deep connection between humans and nature, and how plants have served as spiritual and healing guides over generations. Respecting and honoring these traditions are essential to preserving their cultural and spiritual richness, while also sensitively navigating the path towards greater understanding and dialog between Indigenous cultures and the modern world.

BETWEEN REALITY AND BEYOND REALITY

The philosophical debate about whether psychedelic substances expand consciousness has been an exciting and often controversial topic of discussion in academic, scientific, and spiritual circles. At the heart of this debate lies the fundamental question of whether psychedelic-induced experiences broaden human consciousness or simply modify sensory perception.

Proponents of the idea that psychedelic substances expand consciousness argue that these substances have the potential to push individuals beyond the daily limits of perception and cognition. They argue that psychedelic experiences can open doors to deep levels of introspection, self-discovery, and connection with spiritual dimensions. Through altered perception, they argue that people can access mental states and perspectives that are normally beyond their reach in ordinary consciousness. From this perspective, psychedelic substances are seen as tools to transcend the conventional limitations of the mind and experience a broader and deeper reality.

On the other hand, skeptics argue that what psychedelic substances do is alter perception and create illusions rather than expand true consciousness.

From this perspective, psychedelic experiences can be influenced by altered neurological patterns and sensory distortions, leading to subjective interpretations and perceptions that do not necessarily translate into a deeper understanding or a genuine increase in consciousness. They question whether these experiences are merely manifestations of altered brain processes, and whether the supposed "revelations" are more than ephemeral.

This debate also opens the door to deeper explorations of the very nature of consciousness and reality. Proponents of expanding consciousness argue that psychedelic experiences can provide glimpses of dimensions of reality that are normally hidden from our limited perception. They argue that human consciousness is inherently limited, and that psychedelic substances can act as catalysts to unlock otherwise inaccessible aspects of reality.

From a more philosophical point of view, the question arises whether consciousness itself is a subjective construction based on our sensory perceptions and limited by our cognitive structures. Do psychedelic substances really expand consciousness or simply open temporary windows into alternative ways of perceiving and experiencing reality?

Moreover, the debate on the expansion of consciousness is intertwined with concepts of spirituality and transcendence. Some argue that psychedelic experiences can provide direct access to states of consciousness that resemble mystical and spiritual experiences, leading to connection with a higher or divine reality. Others may argue that these experiences are simply products of brain chemistry and lack a genuine connection to the transcendental.

The debate is intertwined with broader philosophical questions about the nature of consciousness and perception. What constitutes a truly expanded experience of consciousness? Is it possible to transcend human limitation and access a wider and deeper reality through chemicals? Or are these experiences simply a reflection of altered neurological activity without real involvement in the expansion of consciousness?

EXPLANATION OF HOW MICRODOSES WORK IN THE BODY AND MIND

Microdoses, despite their small size, have a surprisingly subtle but significant impact on the human body and mind. Its mode of operation is intricate and multifaceted, based on interactions between active compounds and biological systems. Although the mechanisms behind microdoses are still being fully explored, some key processes that could explain how they influence human experience have been identified.

Neurotransmitters and Neuronal Plasticity:

One of the main pathways through which microdoses can exert their effects is through the modulation of neurotransmitters, the chemical messengers of the brain. Compounds such as psilocybin and LSD, for example, seem to interact with serotonin receptors, which play an essential role in regulating mood, sleep, and other cognitive processes. These interactions may influence the release and reabsorption of serotonin, which in turn may have an impact on emotional and mental well-being.

In addition, microdoses also seem to influence neuronal plasticity, the ability of the brain to form new connections and adapt to new experiences. This may explain why some people report improvements in creativity, concentration, and problem solving after microdosing. Active compounds could facilitate communication between different brain regions and stimulate the formation of new neural networks.

Modulation of Cerebral Blood Flow:

Microdoses can also affect cerebral blood flow, which in turn may influence cognition and perception. Some studies suggest that microdoses may increase blood flow to specific areas of the brain, which may be related to increased mental clarity and increased neuronal plasticity.

Reducing Ego Activity and Self-Awareness:

Another interesting aspect is the possible reduction of the activity of the "ego", the sense of identity and self-awareness. Some users report a sense of greater connection to their environment and a decreased focus on themselves. This decline in ego activity may be related to greater openness to innovative ideas, perspectives, and emotions.

Dopamine and Glutamate receptors:

Other compounds present in microdoses could interact with neurotransmitter receptors such as dopamine and glutamate, which are related to reward, pleasure, and cognition. These interactions could contribute to the emotional and cognitive effects reported by users.

Synchronization and Brain Connectivity:

Microdoses can also affect brain connectivity and the synchronization of neural networks. Some studies suggest that psychedelic compounds may improve communication between different brain regions that typically do not interact as much. This could lead to greater integration of information and a more holistic experience of reality.

Reducing Mind Control System Activity:

Another intriguing aspect is how microdoses might reduce the activity of the "mind control system." This is the part of the brain that is involved in self-evaluation, concern for the future and the past, and self-reflection. Reducing this activity could contribute to a greater sense of being present in the moment and less rumination on past or future concerns.

Interaction with Synaptic Plasticity:

It has been hypothesized that microdoses could interact with synaptic plasticity, which is the ability of connections between neurons to change in response to experience. This could have implications for the way we learn and reconfigure our emotional responses.

It is important to note that the way microdoses interact with the body and mind can vary depending on the substance used, dose, individual sensitivity, and other factors. Moreover, research in this area is ongoing and continues to shed light on the mechanisms behind these subtle but significant experiences.

Microdoses seem to influence a number of neurochemical and neural processes in the human body and mind. Although more research is needed to fully understand all the mechanisms involved, these small doses have the potential to trigger subtle but powerful changes in perception, mood, and cognition. Its functioning is an exciting and constantly evolving topic at the intersection of science, therapy, and self-exploration.

Microdoses are exciting territory in which science, medicine and self-exploration converge. As more research accumulates and these mechanisms are better understood, we are likely to gain a fuller understanding of how these small doses can influence our mind, body, and life experience.

COMPARISON WITH OTHER THERAPEUTIC APPROACHES AND TRADITIONAL MEDICINE

Microdoses represent a unique therapeutic approach in the landscape of mental health and wellbeing. Comparing them with other therapeutic approaches and traditional medicine provides a more complete view of its benefits and limitations.

Conventional therapies, such as cognitive-behavioral therapy (CBT) and prescription drug use, have been used for decades to address a variety of mental disorders. These approaches are based on psychology, neuroscience, and pharmacology, and have proven effective in many cases. Unlike microdoses, conventional therapies do not involve ingestion of psychoactive substances. Instead, they rely on conversation, learning coping strategies, and chemically adjusting the brain with drugs.

Traditional medicine, encompassing a variety of cultural practices and belief systems, has also incorporated natural substances for therapeutic purposes for centuries. However, substances used in traditional medicine are often not administered in subperceptual doses as in microdoses, but may be consumed in more significant amounts or used in ceremonial rituals. Microdoses represent a convergence between traditional medicine and modern science by exploring how substances can have subtle effects and therapeutic benefits in smaller doses.

Microdoses are often used as tools for self-examination and personal growth. Unlike many conventional therapeutic approaches that focus on treating specific disorders, microdoses can be applied by individuals interested in improving their general well-being, increasing creativity, and gaining a deeper understanding of themselves. This more holistic approach aligns with the current movement toward promoting mental health and wellbeing rather than simply addressing the disease.

Instead of seeing microdoses as a replacement for other therapeutic approaches, many people see them as a complementary tool that can be integrated with conventional therapies, mindfulness, yoga, and other methods. Microdoses can provide new perspectives and trigger profound experiences that can then be explored in a therapeutic setting.

One of the biggest challenges with microdoses is the lack of regulation and limited knowledge about their long-term effects. Compared to conventional therapies and prescription drugs, microdoses may lack the same amount of research and clinical data. This makes it important for those who consider microdoses as part of their therapeutic approach to adopt an informed and responsible approach.

One of the key differences between microdoses and some conventional therapeutic approaches is personalization. Microdoses tend to be more personalized in terms of dose and frequency of use. Individuals may adjust their microdose regimen according to their sensitivity, goals, and personal responses. In contrast, some conventional therapies may follow a more standardized approach due to established protocols and dosing guidelines.

Microdoses and many conventional therapeutic approaches differ in their approach to addressing mental health problems. While microdoses can help address the underlying causes and triggers of emotional problems, some conventional therapeutic approaches focus on relieving specific symptoms. This makes microdoses attractive to those who wish to explore and address the deep roots of their emotional challenges.

Microdoses can promote deep introspection and self-awareness. This can be beneficial for those seeking to understand their thinking patterns, emotions, and behaviors. On the other hand, many conventional therapeutic approaches focus on providing patients with specific tools and strategies to address their problems and improve their daily functioning.

One significant difference is the level of scientific evidence and regulation supporting each approach. Conventional therapeutic approaches generally have stronger clinical research support and are regulated by health agencies. Microdoses, although gaining attention and increasing evidence, still face challenges in terms of rigorous research and official recognition.

It is important to consider the role of expectations and the placebo effect in both approaches. Both microdoses and conventional therapies can generate positive results due to the expectations and beliefs of the individual. Personal perception and interaction with the therapist or substance can influence outcomes.

The choice between microdoses, conventional therapeutic approaches, and traditional medicine depends on personal preferences, individual needs, and the orientation of medical care. Some people may find value in combining various approaches, while others may resonate more deeply with a particular approach. The most important thing is to take an informed approach and consult with health care practitioners before making decisions about mental health and well-being.

COMMON SUBSTANCES IN MICRODOSES

EXPLORING THE KEYS TO SMALL-SCALE TRANSFORMATION

In the previous chapter, we unravel the foundations of microdoses and their position at the crossroads between traditional and alternative medicine. Now, we venture to the next level of our journey: the very substances that form the core of microdoses. In this chapter, we will examine closely a wide range of compounds, some of natural and other manufactured origin, which are used in the practice of microdoses.

From ancient civilizations to the modern era, humanity has explored plants, minerals, and compounds in the hope of finding the key to altered perception, deep introspection, and inner healing. The substances that we consider in this chapter are both known for their psychedelic properties and for their subtle effects not discernible to the naked eye. Each has its own history, its own chemistry, and its own interaction with the human body.

We will unravel the properties and potential benefits of the most common substances in microdoses. From psychedelic classics like LSD and psilocybin to lesser-known compounds like cannabis and other herbs microdosing, we will approach each with an open mind and a scientific focus. What makes these substances so powerful at such small doses? How can they influence the brain and nervous system so profoundly?

We will explore the potential effects of these substances in a variety of areas, from improving mood and creativity to reducing stress and anxiety. We will also investigate how microdoses could have therapeutic applications and how some of these substances have been studied in the context of mental health disorders.

In addition to examining the individual properties of each substance, we will address the practical and ethical considerations that accompany its use in the form of microdoses. How are they dosed safely? What are the risks and precautions associated with their use? What role does legality play in this equation?

As we delve into the common substances in microdoses, I invite readers to maintain a balance between fascination and responsibility. Exploration for these substances can be transformative, but it also requires an informed and conscious approach.

Join us in this exploration of the keys to small-scale transformation, as we unveil the secrets these substances hold and how they can offer unique perspectives on the journey of self-reflection and wellbeing.

DESCRIPTION OF NON-PSYCHEDELIC SUBSTANCES

Although microdoses are often associated with psychedelic substances such as LSD or psilocybin, nonpsychedelic substances are also used in this practice with the aim of improving well-being, concentration, and creativity. These substances are chosen for their ability to influence certain aspects of the body and mind without inducing significant psychedelic effects.

We will now list and briefly describe some of these substances:

1. Caffeine microdose:

Caffeine is one of the most widely consumed substances in the world. In the form of coffee, tea or supplements, caffeine is used in microdoses to increase energy, improve concentration and alertness. In exceedingly small doses, caffeine can stimulate the central nervous system without generating noticeable psychedelic effects.

2. Lion's Mane (Hericium erinaceus) microdose:

Lion's Mane is a medicinal mushroom that has been associated with benefits for brain function and nervous system health. Compounds in this fungus, such as perinacin and hericenone, are thought to stimulate nerve growth and brain plasticity. Lion's Mane microdoses are used in the pursuit of greater mental clarity and cognitive improvement.

3. Bacopa monnieri microdose:

This is an extract from a traditional plant used in Ayurvedic medicine. Bacopa monnieri is thought to improve memory and cognitive function by affecting neurotransmitters and neuronal plasticity. Microdoses of Bacopa monnieri are used to promote brain health and mental performance.

4. Rhodiola rosea microdose:

Rhodiola rosea is an adaptogenic plant that has been linked to improved stress resistance, mood, and energy. In microdoses, it seeks to increase resistance to stress and improve cognitive function without generating significant alterations in perception.

5. Ashwagandha microdose:

Another popular adaptogen, Ashwagandha, has been used in Ayurvedic medicine for centuries. In microdoses, it is believed that Ashwagandha can help reduce anxiety, improve mood, and promote relaxation without causing psychedelic effects.

6. Ginkgo biloba microdose:

Ginkgo biloba is a plant known for its potential to improve blood circulation and cognitive function. Compounds in Ginkgo biloba are thought to increase cerebral blood flow and protect nerve cells. Ginkgo biloba microdoses are used to improve memory and concentration.

7. L-Theanine microdose:

L-theanine is an amino acid present in green tea and has been associated with promoting relaxation and stress reduction without causing drowsiness. In micro dosage, L-theanine is used to improve focus and mental clarity, as well as to reduce anxiety.

8. CBD (Cannabidiol) microdose:

CBD is a non-psychedelic component of cannabis that has gained popularity for its potential benefits in reducing anxiety and stress, as well as in relieving pain and improving sleep. In microdoses, CBD can be used for its relaxing and potentially anxiolytic effects without inducing psychotropic effects.

9. Piracetam microdose:

Nootropic drugs such as piracetam are used in microdoses to improve cognitive function and memory. Piracetam and other nootropics can influence neurotransmitters and synaptic plasticity to potentially improve concentration and information retention.

10. Modafinil microdose:

Modafinil is a prescription drug used to treat excessive sleepiness and narcolepsy. In microdoses, it has been used to increase alertness, concentration, and mental energy. However, because of its stimulating nature, it should be used with caution and under medical supervision.

POTENTIAL BENEFITS OF CAFFEINE

Microdosing caffeine involves taking a tiny amount of the substance, usually less than the amount in a standard cup of coffee. Unlike other psychedelic microdoses that focus on changing perception and awareness, caffeine microdoses are aimed at increasing mental and physical activity as well as improving focusing ability and productivity.

Proponents of caffeine microdoses argue that it can have positive effects in terms of cognitive improvement, increased energy, and reduced fatigue. It is suggested that it may be particularly useful in situations where sustained focus and mental performance are required, such as in demanding work or academic environments. In addition, the caffeine microdose can also be seen as an alternative to higher doses of caffeine that can cause nervousness or restlessness.

Although caffeine is widely consumed and accepted in society, it is essential to consider the challenges and risks associated with its microdose. Because caffeine is a potent stimulant, even in small doses, it can have side effects such as insomnia, nervousness, and increased heart rate. Caffeine dependence and tolerance are also important considerations, as regular consumption can lead to reduced sensitivity to its effects.

Exploring the potential effects and benefits of caffeine microdosing offers a unique perspective in the field of cognitive optimization and performance improvement. Although not related to psychedelic experiences in the traditional sense, the caffeine microdose reflects how substances can be used strategically to improve specific aspects of mental and physical function in modern life. However, it is essential that people consider their own sensitivities, needs and goals when considering the microdose of caffeine, and that they seek professional guidance if they are looking to optimize their intake in a healthy and balanced way.

POTENTIAL BENEFITS OF LION'S MANE (HERICIUM ERINACEUS)

Lion's Mane is an edible mushroom that has been revered in traditional Asian medicine for centuries due to its alleged ability to improve brain function and promote nervous health.

Instead of affecting consciousness and perception as psychedelic substances do, Lion's Mane microdose focuses on its neuroprotective and potentially neuronal growth-stimulating properties. Lion's Mane has been shown to contain bioactive compounds, such as erinacines and hericenones, that can promote the synthesis of nerve growth factors and stimulate the development of new brain cells. These effects may result in improvements in memory, cognition, mental clarity, and nervous system function.

Lion's Mane microdoses could have benefits in terms of cognitive optimization and mitigation of age-related cognitive impairment. In addition, some initial studies have also indicated possible positive effects in reducing stress and anxiety, which could make this approach an attractive option for those seeking to improve their emotional and mental well-being.

POTENTIAL BENEFITS OF BACOPA MONNIERI

Unlike psychedelic substances that alter perception and consciousness, Bacopa monnieri microdose focuses on its potential to increase cognition and reduce the effects of stress on the body and mind. Active compounds present in Bacopa monnieri, such as bacosides, are thought to have positive effects on memory, concentration, and overall brain function. In addition, it has been suggested that Bacopa monnieri can function as an adaptogen, helping the body manage stress and promoting a general balance in the nervous system.

Microdoses of Bacopa monnieri may have benefits in terms of cognitive improvement, reduction of mental fatigue, and support of emotional well-being. Some initial studies have indicated that Bacopa monnieri may have promising effects on long-term memory and overall brain function. In addition, its ability to reduce stress could make this practice an attractive option for those seeking to better manage the demands of modern life.

POTENTIAL BENEFITS OF RHODIOLA ROSEA

Rhodiola rosea microdoses focus on its ability to influence stress regulation and mood improvement. It is believed that active plant compounds, such as rosavin and salicrosides, can influence the body's response to stress by regulating the nervous and hormonal systems. This could translate into reduced fatigue, increased stress resistance, and improved ability to cope with the challenges of daily life.

Proponents of Rhodiola rosea's microdose argue that it could have benefits in terms of improving mood, reducing anxiety, and supporting mental clarity. It is suggested that Rhodiola rosea can help increase emotional resilience and improve concentration, which could make this practice an attractive option for those looking for a natural approach to dealing with stress and improving their mental well-being.

POTENTIAL BENEFITS OF ASHWAGANDHA

It is believed that the active ingredients of Ashwagandha can influence hormonal and neurochemical regulation, which could result in reduced stress, anxiety, and fatigue. In addition, it has been suggested that Ashwagandha could have positive effects on cognitive function and sleep quality.

Ashwagandha could have benefits in terms of improved mood, reduced anxiety, and support for mental clarity. It is suggested that Ashwagandha can help increase stress resilience and improve concentration, which could make this practice an attractive option for those looking to improve their emotional well-being and ability to manage the demands of modern life.

POTENTIAL BENEFITS OF GINKGO BILOBA

The exploration of the effects and potential benefits of the Ginkgo biloba microdose delves into the realm of medicinal plants with centuries of use in traditional medicine, in this case, in Chinese and Asian culture. Ginkgo biloba, known for its distinctive leaf shape and longevity as a species, has been prized for its potential benefits for brain and circulatory health.

Unlike psychedelic substances that alter perception, the Ginkgo biloba microdose focuses on its supposed effects on improving blood circulation and cognitive function. It is believed that flavonoids and terpenoids present in Ginkgo biloba can have positive effects on the dilation of blood vessels and on the protection of nerve cells from oxidative damage. This could translate into improvements in memory, concentration, and cognitive performance.

Proponents of Ginkgo biloba microdose argue that it could have benefits in terms of brain optimization, increased mental clarity, and support for circulatory health. It is suggested that Ginkgo biloba can influence cognitive function and protect the brain from the effects of aging and oxidative stress, which could make this practice an attractive option for those seeking to improve their brain function and mental well-being.

POTENTIAL BENEFITS OF L-THEANINE

L-Theanine microdoses focus on its ability to influence neurotransmission and modulation of brain activity. It has been suggested that L-Theanine may promote the production of neurotransmitters such as serotonin and dopamine, which are related to mood regulation and sense of well-being. In addition, L-Theanine has also been associated with promoting relaxation and stress reduction.

Proponents of L-Theanine microdose argue that it could have benefits in terms of improving mood, reducing anxiety, and supporting concentration. It is suggested that L-Theanine can have a calming effect without causing drowsiness, which could make this practice an attractive option for those looking to manage stress and improve their emotional and mental well-being.

POTENTIAL BENEFITS OF CBD (CANNABIDIOL)

Exploring the potential effects and benefits of CBD (Cannabidiol) microdose immerses us in the world of cannabinoids and their relationship to mental health and physical well-being. CBD, one of the main compounds present in the cannabis plant, has gained attention in recent years due to its possible effects in reducing stress, anxiety, and pain, without causing the psychoactive effects associated with THC (tetrahydrocannabinol).

CBD focuses on its ability to influence the endocannabinoid system, a regulatory system found throughout the body and related to homeostasis and regulation of various physiological functions. It has been suggested that CBD can have anti-inflammatory, anxiolytic and analgesic effects by interacting with cannabinoid receptors in the body.

CBD may have benefits in terms of reducing anxiety, improving sleep, and relieving pain. It is suggested that CBD can influence the function of the nervous system and help regulate responses to stress, which could make this practice an attractive option for those looking for a natural alternative to manage their mental and physical health challenges.

POTENTIAL BENEFITS OF PIRACETAM

Piracetam focuses on its ability to influence neurotransmission and synaptic plasticity in the brain. It is suggested that Piracetam may increase the amount of oxygen and glucose available to brain cells, which may result in an improvement in cognitive function and in the ability to process information.

Proponents of Piracetam microdosing argue that it could have benefits in terms of increased concentration, improved information retention, and increased mental energy. It is suggested that Piracetam can optimize neuronal activity and promote communication between brain cells, which could make this practice an attractive option for those seeking to improve their cognitive function and performance in intellectual tasks.

POTENTIAL BENEFITS OF MODAFINIL

Modafinil as a stimulant medicine has an impact on wakefulness and cognition. Modafinil is a prescription drug used to treat excessive sleepiness associated with sleep disorders such as narcolepsy and sleep apnea, and has gained some popularity for its supposed ability to improve concentration and mental alertness.

Modafinil focuses on its influence on central nervous system activity and brain neurochemistry. Modafinil is thought to increase levels of neurotransmitters such as dopamine, which could result in increased wakefulness and improved cognitive function, including attention, memory and learning ability.

Modafinil may have benefits in terms of increased mental energy, increased cognitive clarity, and improved productivity. It is suggested that Modafinil can help overcome fatigue and maintain a constant state of alertness, which could make this practice an attractive option for those looking to improve their performance in tasks that require attention and prolonged concentration.

DESCRIPTION OF PSYCHEDELIC SUBSTANCES

Psychedelic substances used in microdoses are those that, in subperceptual doses, can induce subtle effects on the mind and body without causing the full psychedelic experiences associated with higher doses.

These substances are chosen for their potential therapeutic, creative, and self-exploration benefits. Here is a description of some psychedelic substances typically used in microdoses:

1. LSD (lysergic acid diethylamide):

LSD is a psychedelic substance known for its mind- and perception-altering effects. In microdosing, LSD is thought to increase creativity, concentration, and mood. Microdoses of LSD have been reported to produce an increase in energy and mental clarity without causing significant visual hallucinations.

2. Psilocybin (Magic Mushrooms):

Psilocybin mushrooms contain psilocybin, a compound that can induce psychedelic experiences. In microdoses, psilocybin can increase introspection, creativity, and emotional openness. Psilocybin microdoses are thought to influence cognition, mood, and perception subtly.

3. MDMA (3,4-methylenedioxymethamphetamine):

Although not considered strictly psychedelic, MDMA is a substance that can have emotional openness and empathy effects. In microdoses, the aim is to promote emotional connection and improve mood. Microdoses of MDMA are thought to influence interpersonal communication and emotional self-examination.

4. DMT (Dimethyltryptamine):

DMT is known for its intense psychedelic nature in full doses. In microdoses, it is believed that DMT can generate an increase in creativity and spiritual outlook. However, due to its potent nature, DMT microdosing should be done with extreme caution and under appropriate supervision.

5. Mescaline (from the San Pedro and Peyote Cactus):

Mescaline is a compound present in certain psychedelic cactus such as San Pedro and Peyote. In microdoses, it is believed that mescaline can induce states of greater introspection, spirituality, and connection with nature. Microdoses of mescaline are used to explore spirituality and self-awareness.

6. 2C-B (2,5-dimethoxy-4-bromophenylethylamine):

2C-B is a psychedelic compound that belongs to the family of phenylethylamines. In full doses, it may induce psychedelic visual and emotional effects. In microdosing, 2C-B is thought to increase energy, improve mood, and enhance creativity. Due to its potency, microdosing with 2C-B should be performed with caution and monitoring.

7. LSD Microdot (LSD Pill Microdose):

Apart from LSD in liquid or paper form, there are also microdoses of LSD in the form of microdots, small pills that contain subperceptual doses. Microdots are another option for those looking to experience the benefits of LSD microdoses in a more convenient way.

8. Microdoses of Ancestral Fungi and Plants:

In addition to the psilocybin mushrooms, certain plants such as iboga, used in some African spiritual traditions, and ayahuasca, used in indigenous ceremonies in the Amazon, have also been used in microdoses for purposes of self-exploration, spirituality, and connection with nature.

It is essential to remember that psychedelic substances, even in microdoses, can have unpredictable effects and vary by person, dose, and environment. In addition, the legal implications and health risks should be carefully considered. Psychedelic substances are not recommended without adequate medical supervision and a full understanding of the potential risks and benefits.

The choice of using psychedelic substances in microdoses must be made responsibly and educationally. Those interested in exploring the potential benefits of these substances should seek guidance from qualified health care practitioners and consider legal and safety factors before embarking on this practice.

POTENTIAL BENEFITS OF LSD (LYSERGIC ACID DIETHYLAMIDE)

Exploring the potential effects and benefits of Lysergic Acid Diethylamide, better known as LSD, is a topic that has captured the attention of scientists, doctors, and mental health enthusiasts for decades. LSD is a psychedelic substance distinguished by its ability to induce profoundly altered experiences of consciousness and perception. Although historically associated with the counterculture of the 1960s, its therapeutic potential has rekindled interest and research in recent years.

In terms of effects, LSD is known for its ability to generate intense psychedelic experiences. These experiences may include changes in visual perception, distortion of time and space, and greater emotional openness. The substance acts on serotonin receptors in the brain, resulting in a wide range of effects that vary depending on the dose and the environment in which it is consumed. Some people may experience feelings of euphoria and spiritual connection, while others may face episodes of anxiety or paranoia.

In the therapeutic field, LSD has been the target of interest due to its potential to treat conditions such as treatment-resistant depression, terminal anxiety, and post-traumatic stress disorder. It has been theorized that psychedelic experiences induced by LSD could help reconfigure patterns of thought and behavior, offering a new and more adaptable perspective on mental health problems. Some preliminary studies suggest that LSD may be useful in assisted psychedelic therapy, in which the substance is given in a controlled setting and guided by trained therapists.

However, it is important to note that LSD also carries risks and challenges. Their potential to generate intense and sometimes uncontrollable experiences can be problematic, especially in people predisposed to psychotic disorders or in unsupervised settings. Moreover, the legality and stigma surrounding LSD are still significant barriers to its research and therapeutic use in many parts of the world.

In addition, particular attention should be paid to the selection of patients suitable for LSD therapy. It is essential to identify clear criteria for inclusion and exclusion, as well as to thoroughly assess patients' mental health and physical condition before considering their participation in LSD therapies. This will help minimize potential risks and maximize therapeutic benefits.

Another crucial aspect is the creation of safe and supportive environments for LSD administration in a therapeutic environment. Guidance from trained therapists and appropriate structuring of experience are critical to ensuring that patients can productively process and understand their psychedelic experiences. Subsequent preparation and integration also play a vital role in the therapeutic process.

Exploration of the effects and benefits of LSD is a constantly evolving field. While there is preliminary evidence to support its therapeutic potential, more rigorous and controlled research is needed to fully understand how it can be safely and effectively integrated into the medical and therapeutic arena. Ultimately, LSD remains a substance that requires careful exploration and a science-based approach to harness its potential and minimize its risks.

POTENTIAL BENEFITS OF PSILOCYBIN (MAGIC MUSHROOMS)

Psilocybin is a psychedelic substance found in certain fungi, and its use can induce highly altered experiences of consciousness. The effects of magic mushrooms can vary but often include changes in visual perception, altered sense of time, and heightened emotional connection. These effects result from the interaction of psilocybin with serotonin receptors in the brain, triggering a cascade of neurochemical events that result in deeply introspective and enlightening experiences.

One of the most notable potential benefits of psilocybin is its ability to induce mystical or spiritual experiences. These experiences are often described as moments of deep connection with the universe, divinity, or a broader sense of purpose. It has been observed that these experiences can have a lasting impact on the individual's perception of himself, his life, and his place in the world.

From a therapeutic perspective, magic mushrooms have gained attention for their potential in the treatment of conditions such as treatment-resistant depression, anxiety, and post-traumatic stress disorder. Psidocyclin-assisted psychedelic therapy involves giving the substance in a controlled setting and with guidance from trained therapists. Psilocybin-induced psychedelic experiences are thought to help patients cope with and process past trauma, reconfigure negative thinking patterns, and experience greater emotional and cognitive openness.

However, as with any psychedelic substance, magic mushrooms are not without challenges and risks. The intense and sometimes challenging experiences that can arise during a psilocybin trip can be difficult for some people to manage, especially in the absence of proper guidance. Safety and legality are also key considerations, as psilocybin is still banned in many parts of the world.

POTENTIAL BENEFITS OF MDMA (3,4-METHYLENEDIOXYMETHAMPHETAMINE)

From a therapeutic perspective, MOTAPM has generated interest due to its ability to facilitate open communication and emotional connection in the context of therapy. MDMA-assisted therapy involves controlled administration of the substance in a therapeutic setting, usually in couples or small groups, with guidance from trained therapists. It has been observed that MDMA can help patients overcome emotional blockages, past trauma, and difficulties in interpersonal communication.

One of the most prominent potential benefits of MDMA in the therapeutic field is its ability to foster empathy and interpersonal connection. During a MDMA therapy session, patients often experience greater emotional openness to themselves and others. This can be especially valuable in treating conditions such as post-traumatic stress disorder, where connection with others and expression of emotions can be difficult.

However, it is important to address the risks and challenges associated with MOTAPM. Its ability to increase the release of neurotransmitters can have side effects, such as dehydration and stress on the cardiovascular system. In addition, the recreational and unsupervised use of MOTAPM has led to concerns about its safety and legality.

POTENTIAL BENEFITS OF DMT (DIMETHYLTRYPTAMINE)

DMT acts on serotonin receptors in the brain, inducing altered states of consciousness that are often described as "travel". These journeys may vary in the length and nature of lived experiences, but they often include vivid visions, feelings of connection with the divine or the cosmic, and deep introspection. The effects of DMT are known to be extremely powerful and can be both visual and emotional.

From a therapeutic perspective, DMT has begun to receive attention because of its ability to induce profoundly enlightening and transformative experiences. It has been theorized that these experiences can help individuals confront past traumas, change negative thinking patterns, and develop greater emotional and spiritual openness. DMT therapy has been explored in clinical and ceremonial settings, and it has been suggested that it could be especially valuable in the treatment of conditions such as depression, anxiety, and post-traumatic stress disorder.

In addition, legality and safety are crucial considerations when exploring the DMT. Although found in some plants and used in traditional contexts in certain cultures, DMT remains a controlled substance in many parts of the world. Lack of regulation and supervision can increase the risks associated with recreational and non-therapeutic use.

POTENTIAL BENEFITS OF MESCALINE (FROM SAN PEDRO AND PEYOTE CACTUS)

Mescaline has aroused interest because of its potential to facilitate introspection and exploration of thought and behavior patterns. It has been theorized that mescaline-generated experiences can enable individuals to cope with past traumas, understand internal conflicts, and achieve greater mental and emotional clarity. Some advocates of mescaline therapy argue that it may be beneficial in treating conditions such as depression, anxiety, and addiction.

However, addressing the challenges and risks associated with mescaline is essential. Mescaline-induced psychedelic experiences can be intense and challenging for some people, especially in the absence of adequate therapeutic guidance. In addition, legality and access to mescaline vary by region and culture, which may affect individuals' ability to access therapy and research in this field.

Exploring the potential effects and benefits of mescaline is a process that requires a combination of respect for cultural traditions and rigorous scientific evaluation. Although mescaline has been used in spiritual and ceremonial contexts for centuries, its therapeutic potential in the contemporary setting remains the subject of research DMT and debate. Proper integration in therapy, development of safe protocols, and respectful collaboration with Indigenous communities that have maintained these traditions are critical to understanding and harnessing the potential benefits of mescaline in addressing mental health issues and advancing scientific knowledge.

POTENTIAL BENEFITS OF 2C-B (2,5-DIMETHOXY-4-BROMOPHENYLETHYLAMINE)

Exploring the potential effects and benefits of 2C-B, also known as "Nexus" or "Eros", takes us into the world of substituted phenylethylamines, a class of psychedelic substances that have gained interest in psychedelic research and experimentation circles. 2C-B is a compound that belongs to this family and is characterized by its ability to induce unique and distinctive psychedelic experiences.

2C-B acts on the serotonin and dopamine receptors in the brain, resulting in effects that may vary depending on the dose and the context in which it is consumed. It is often described as a substance that combines elements of stimulation, hallucination, and empathy. Effects may include changes in visual perception, greater sensory sensitivity, and greater emotional and sensual openness. Experiences with 2C-B have been observed to be intense and, in many cases, associated with a sense of deep connection with oneself, others and the environment.

In therapeutic terms, 2C-B has become a focus of interest, albeit to a lesser extent than other psychedelic substances. Some therapists and psychedelic enthusiasts believe that its unique properties, such as the combination of hallucinogenic effects and mild stimulants, could be useful in therapeutic contexts. It has been speculated that 2C-B could be used to facilitate communication and introspection in therapy, as well as to address anxiety and stress.

POTENTIAL BENEFITS OF LSD MICRODOT (PILL-SHAPED LSD MICRODOSE)

Unlike conventional doses of LSD, which are taken to induce intense psychedelic experiences, microdosing involves taking an exceedingly small amount of the substance, usually about one-tenth of a standard recreational dose. Proponents of microdosing argue that this approach can have beneficial stimulating and cognitive effects, such as increased concentration, creativity, and positive mood, without the full hallucinogenic effects.

The effects of LSD microdose may vary by person, dose, and context. Some individuals report greater mental clarity, a greater sense of energy, and an improvement in creativity. It has been speculated that microdosing could be useful in work and academic settings, as well as in stress and anxiety management.

POTENTIAL BENEFITS OF ANCESTRAL FUNGI AND PLANTS

Various cultures have used these substances for spiritual and healing purposes throughout history. Fungi and plants, such as peyote, magic mushrooms and ayahuasca, have been revered in different traditions for their ability to induce altered states of consciousness that are believed to provide a deeper insight into reality and a greater understanding of self and the cosmos.

Microdosing of fungi and ancestral plants involves taking subperceptible doses of these substances, which means that complete hallucinogenic effects are not experienced. Unlike complete psychedelic journeys, where the experience can be overwhelming and intense, microdosing aims to provide a subtle level of influence that could lead to increased alertness, empathy and connection with nature and spirituality.

Proponents of microdosing ancestral fungi and plants suggest that there may be benefits in terms of increased creativity, introspection, and mental clarity. In addition, some individuals have reported improvements in their emotional and spiritual well-being, as well as greater connection to their environment and to their own values and purpose in life.

SAFETY AND LEGALITY CONSIDERATIONS FOR SUBSTANCES USED

Despite the potential therapeutic and experiential benefits, it is crucial to understand the risks involved and the legal implications that may arise.

First, psychedelic substances, regardless of their form or amount, can have unpredictable effects on different individuals. Reactions to microdoses can vary widely depending on factors such as genetics, mental and physical health status, the environment, and the dose itself. What might be beneficial to one person could be triggering or problematic to another. Careful consideration of personal health and any medical history is essential before embarking on the microdose.

Safety is also linked to the source of substances used in microdoses. The quality and purity of the substances are crucial factors to ensure a safe and positive experience. Obtaining psychedelic substances from unreliable sources may increase the risk of contamination or adulteration, which could have negative health effects. Finding substances of reliable origin and choosing sources that offer quality assurance is an essential consideration.

From a legal perspective, it is crucial to research and understand laws and regulations in the geographic area in which one is located. Laws relating to psychedelic substances may vary significantly from country to country and, in some cases, even within regions of the same country. Some substances, such as LSD and psilocybin, are classified as controlled substances in many jurisdictions and their possession and use may be illegal. Microdosing of illegal substances could have serious legal consequences.

As interest in microdoses continues to grow, it is critical to promote a culture of responsibility and education. Seeking advice from mental health professionals, psychologists, or psychiatrists is an essential step before embarking on a microdose. These practitioners can provide a personalized assessment and help determine whether microdoses are appropriate and safe in a specific situation.

The path to microdoses must be approached with caution, responsibility, and awareness. While there is anecdotal and emerging evidence to support potential benefits, there is always a need to balance these aspects with potential health and legal risks. Making informed decisions and considering both safety and legality is essential to ensure a positive and healthy experience in the field of microdoses of psychedelic and ancestral substances.

Responsible microdosing practices are essential in the search for a safe experience and potential benefits. This means starting with extremely low doses and increasing gradually only if the effects are well tolerated. Keeping a detailed record of the doses, effects, and emotions experienced can provide valuable information for assessing impact over time.

In addition, the environment in which the microdose is performed plays a crucial role. Choosing a quiet and comfortable environment, preferably in the company of trusted people, can contribute to a positive experience. Avoiding stressful situations or unknown locations during microdosing may minimize the possibility of unwanted emotional responses.

Mentality and intention are also significant elements in microdoses. Rather than seeking concrete answers, it was valuable to approach microdoses with openness and curiosity. Being willing to explore one's own thoughts, emotions, and behavioral patterns can facilitate greater self-knowledge and personal growth.

In relation to legality, it is imperative to investigate and understand the current regulations in their location. Some countries and states are moving toward decriminalizing or legalizing certain psychedelic substances for therapeutic purposes, while elsewhere, use and possession can have serious legal consequences. Keeping informed about any changes in legislation is essential to making informed decisions.

HALLUCINOGENIC MUSHROOMS

In the vast realm of nature, certain fungi possess the astonishing power to alter human perception, triggering psychedelic experiences that have intrigued humanity throughout history. This chapter will immerse us in the fascinating world of hallucinogenic mushrooms, exploring some of the most notable varieties and their impacts on health and wellbeing. From the iconic Psilocybe cubensis to the mystical Amanita muscaria and the discrete Panaeolus cyanescens, each species reveals a unique set of characteristics, chemical properties, and cultural connections.

The journey begins by unraveling the mysteries of the Psilocybe cubensis, whose roots are intertwined with ancient shamanic traditions and practices. From its origins in tropical climates to its global presence, we will explore its effects on human consciousness and its therapeutic potential. As we move forward, we come across the Psilocybe semilanceata, the "Dwarf Mushroom," whose elegant form and cultural associations offer a unique perspective on the world of hallucinogenic mushrooms.

We will take a leap towards the Amanita muscaria, the "Flyswatter", a species wrapped in mythology and rich in intriguing chemical compounds. From its red and white hat to its effects on the mind, we will explore its cultural history and its possible therapeutic applications. Finally, we will delve into the realm of the Panaeolus cyanescens, the "Blue Meanies", whose small size hides powerful psychoactive properties and arouses questions about the ethics and safety of their consumption.

Through this journey, we will seek to understand not only the botanical and chemical aspects of these hallucinogenic mushrooms, but also their connections to spirituality, mythology, and the human mind. From grasslands to forests, these varieties invite us to explore the intersection between nature and consciousness, raising compelling questions about the limits of perception and the potential health benefits and risks. Prepare to immerse yourself in a world where science and tradition meet, where the boundaries of reality blur, and where understanding these hallucinogenic mushrooms invites us on a journey of knowledge and discovery.

PSILOCYBE CUBENSIS

Psilocybe cubensis, also known as "magic mushrooms" or "psilocybin mushrooms", are one of the most well-known and widely distributed species of hallucinogenic mushrooms. Originating mainly in tropical and subtropical regions, these mushrooms have gained their popularity due to the psychoactive compounds they contain, mainly psilocybin and psilocine.

Psilocybe cubensis have an origin that goes back to places like South America, Mexico, and other areas with warm and humid climates. Despite their roots in these regions, these mushrooms have proven adaptable and have been found in various parts of the world, including parts of Asia, Africa, and Australia. Its ability to thrive in different environments has contributed to its global accessibility.

These mushrooms have a number of distinctive features that make them easily recognizable. Its hat, which can vary in color from white to light brown, has a bell shape that expands as the mushroom ripens. The margin of the hat tends to be lighter, and occasionally, it has remnants of a partial veil that detaches as the mushroom grows.

Throughout history, Psilocybe cubensis have played a significant role in various Indigenous cultures, especially in Latin America. These mushrooms have often been linked to ritual ceremonies and spiritual practices, where they were believed to facilitate communication with the divine and provide transcendental knowledge. This cultural aspect has contributed to the contemporary perception of these mushrooms as tools for the expansion of consciousness and introspection.

Psilocybe cubensis contain psychoactive compounds, psilocybin and psilocybin being the most prominent. These compounds interact with serotoninergic receptors in the brain, triggering psychedelic effects that include altered perception, mood changes, and intensified sensory experiences. The unique combination of these compounds gives these mushrooms their ability to induce psychedelic experiences.

PSILOCYBE SEMILANCEATA (DWARF MUSHROOM)

Psilocybe semilanceata, colloquially known as the "Dwarf Mushroom" or "Liberty Cap", is a variety of hallucinogenic fungus that has captured the attention of both mycological enthusiasts and those interested in the psychoactive properties of mushrooms. This particular species has left a distinctive mark on popular culture, thanks to its unique shape and psychedelic effects.

The Psilocybe semilanceata features a conical hat that narrows to the top, often taking on a shape reminiscent of a cane or spear, hence its scientific name. Its color ranges from brown tones to lighter shades, and its size is generally modest, which contributes to its discretion in natural environments. This fungus usually grows on grasslands, especially those associated with the presence of certain types of pasture.

Throughout history, Psilocybe semilanceata has been the subject of experiences reported by those who have had encounters with it. Narratives include descriptions of intense visual effects, alterations in the perception of time, and a greater appreciation of the surrounding nature. Despite its popularity in recreational culture, scientific studies have shown a growing interest in the therapeutic potential of psychoactive compounds present in this fungus, particularly psilocybin.

What distinguishes Psilocybe semilanceata is the presence of psychoactive compounds, mainly psilocybin and psilocybin. These compounds interact with serotonergic receptors in the brain, triggering psychedelic experiences that can vary in intensity. The unique combination of these compounds gives this mushroom its ability to induce altered states of consciousness, and its chemical profile differentiates it from other varieties of hallucinogenic fungi.

Compared to other hallucinogenic mushrooms, Psilocybe semilanceata stands out for its presence in specific regions and its relationship with certain types of grasslands. Although it shares similarities in terms of psychoactive compounds with other species, its distinctive appearance and specific habitat make it unique in the world of hallucinogenic mushrooms.

AMANITA MUSCARIA (FLYSWATTER)

Amanita muscaria, commonly known as "Fly Agaric" or "Fly Agaric", is a kind of hallucinogenic fungus that has captured the imagination of diverse cultures throughout history. Its distinctive appearance, marked by a bright red hat dotted with white spots, makes it easily recognizable and has contributed to its notoriety in mythology and literature.

This variety of this hallucinogenic mushroom has played a significant role in the mythologies of various cultures. From Siberian to Scandinavian traditions, Amanita muscaria has been associated with shamanic rituals and mystical figures. In some accounts, it is believed that this mushroom had divine properties, being used as a bridge between the spiritual and the earthly world.

Amanita muscaria contains unique active compounds, such as ibotenic acid and muscimol. These compounds interact with the central nervous system, inducing psychoactive effects ranging from euphoria to sensory distortion. Despite its hallucinogenic properties, caution is essential, as it can also have toxic effects if not managed properly.

The look of Amanita muscaria is unmistakable: a deep red convex hat with white spots that evoke images of fairy tales. It usually grows in association with coniferous trees, forming a symbiosis that contributes to its distribution in temperate and boreal areas of the northern hemisphere. This mushroom has been sighted in forests in Europe, Asia, North America, and parts of South America.

Unlike other hallucinogenic mushrooms, Amanita muscaria stands out for its striking appearance and its associations with mythology. Although it shares certain psychoactive compounds with other varieties, such as psilocybin and psilocine, its unique chemical profile confers distinctive properties and effects that may differ in intensity and nature.

It is crucial to approach Amanita muscaria with caution because of its potential toxicity. Inadequate intake can lead to adverse symptoms, including nausea, vomiting, and delirium. However, some studies have explored its possible therapeutic benefits, suggesting that certain compounds present may have applications in the treatment of neuropsychiatric disorders, although more research is needed to confirm these findings.

PANAEOLUS CYANESCENS

Panaeolus cyanescens, commonly known as "Copelandia cyanescens" or "Blue Meanies", is a variety of this hallucinogenic mushroom that has attracted the attention of mycology enthusiasts and consciousness explorers. This particular species stands out for its psychoactive properties and its presence in diverse environments, from grasslands to areas of manure, revealing its ability to thrive under specific conditions.

The Panaeolus cyanescens are characterized by their small size and their hue that varies between brown and beige. Although its appearance may be discrete, its distinctive feature is the ability to develop a blue dye in certain parts when handled or cut, a phenomenon attributed to the presence of chemical compounds reactive to oxygen. This color change has intrigued scholars and contributed to their nickname, "Blue Meanies".

Originally from tropical and subtropical regions, Panaeolus cyanescens are found in a variety of locations around the world. They prefer nutrient-rich habitats, such as well-fertilized grasslands or areas of livestock manure. Their adaptability to different climatic conditions and their ability to grow in different substrates make them a relatively common species in certain ecosystems.

Like other hallucinogenic mushrooms, Panaeolus cyanescens contain psychoactive compounds, psilocybin and psilocybin being the most notable. These compounds interact with serotoninergic receptors in the brain, triggering psychedelic experiences that include changes in perception, alterations in thought, and intensified emotional connections. The variability in the severity of these events may be influenced by factors such as dosage and individual sensitivity.

Although these mushrooms have not been as prominent in cultural and shamanic traditions as other varieties, they have been used by Indigenous communities in certain regions for ritual and spiritual purposes. However, access to and consumption of these mushrooms raise ethical and legal issues in many places, which has led to discussions around their recreational and therapeutic use.

RESEARCH AND EVIDENCE

EXPLORING THE FOUNDATIONS OF KNOWLEDGE ABOUT MICRODOSES

In the previous chapters, we have immersed our minds in the fundamentals of microdoses and explored the substances that make up their essence. Now, it is time to approach with critical and scientific lenses one of the most essential aspects of this topic: the research and empirical evidence supporting the claims and potential of microdoses.

In this chapter, we will embark on a journey of discovery in which we will examine the panorama of scientific studies that have shed light on microdoses. What does research say about the effects of these tiny doses on the human mind and body? What areas have shown promising potential, and where clarity is still lacking?

From controlled clinical studies to research in the field of neuroscience and psychology, we will travel a diverse spectrum of disciplines to assess the validity and reliability of the evidence surrounding microdoses. We will analyze the methods used in these studies, their limitations and how they can influence the way we interpret their results.

In addition to scientific studies, we will also address the importance of empirical evidence. The subjective experiences and testimonials of individuals who have experienced microdoses firsthand play a crucial role in building a holistic understanding. But we must also consider how to balance these narratives with scientific rigor in order to get a complete and accurate picture.

This chapter is not only about reviewing existing evidence, but also about recognizing areas where research is insufficient or at an early stage. Identifying knowledge limitations and gaps is essential for advancing the field of microdoses in a responsible and ethical manner.

Adopt a critical and curious mindset. Scientific research and empirical evidence are the foundation on which any practice or approach is built. By exploring current research and its implications, we will be better equipped to make informed decisions about microdoses, understand their real potential, and embrace a science-based approach to this intriguing and ever-evolving practice.

SUMMARY OF SCIENTIFIC STUDIES AND RESEARCH ON MICRODOSES

As interest in microdoses of psychedelic and ancestral substances has increased, scientific research in this field has gained momentum. While microdose studies are still limited and mostly exploratory, they have shed light on the possible effects and benefits that these small doses could have on people's mental and emotional health.

Most studies have focused on substances such as LSD and psilocybin, and have investigated how microdoses can influence cognition, creativity, emotional perception, and overall mental health. Findings have been mixed, but most suggest that microdoses may have positive effects in terms of subtle improvements in cognition, concentration, and mood. In addition, some studies have reported an increase in creativity and cognitive flexibility in individuals who participated in microdoses.

Regarding mental health, there has been preliminary research suggesting that microdoses could have a positive effect on anxiety and depression. Some anecdotal reports and pilot studies have noted that people who performed microdoses experienced a decrease in the symptoms of these conditions. However, it is critical to note that these results are still preliminary and that stronger research is needed to fully understand the potential therapeutic benefits.

Neuroscience has also begun to address the issue of microdoses, investigating how psychedelic substances can affect brain activity at lower doses. Brain imaging studies have shown changes in brain connectivity and communication between brain regions, suggesting that microdoses could influence the way our brain processes information and emotional experiences.

Importantly, most microdose studies are small, and research methodology and protocols can vary widely. In addition, the scientific community is still working to fully understand the mechanisms of action and potential risks associated with microdoses. More rigorous, large-scale research is needed to confirm and refine current findings.

Scientific studies on microdoses of psychedelic and ancestral substances are at an early but promising stage. Although the results so far have been encouraging in terms of possible improvements in cognition, creativity, and mental health, deeper and more thorough research is needed to fully understand the potential effects and benefits of microdoses.

CRITICAL ANALYSIS OF THE QUALITY AND RELIABILITY OF THE AVAILABLE EVIDENCE

When examining the quality and reliability of the available evidence on microdoses of psychedelic and ancestral substances, it is essential to recognize that most studies in this field are still limited in terms of sample size, experimental design, and rigorous methodology. While there has been an increase in research in recent years, it is important to approach the findings with caution and consider the inherent limitations.

First, much of the existing evidence is based on anecdotal reports and pilot studies with small, unrepresentative samples. These reports may provide interesting insights into individual experiences, but they lack the rigor and control needed to establish reliable causal correlations. The variability in reported effects and the lack of control groups in many of these studies limit the ability to generalize the results to the general population.

In addition, the absence of double-blind, placebo-controlled studies in the field of microdoses is a significant limitation. The lack of a control group and the difficulty of anonymity due to the nature of psychedelic substances may influence the interpretation of the results. Placebo effects and individual expectations may play a key role in the perception of the effects of microdosing.

The lack of a clear consensus on the definition of "microdose" also complicates the interpretation of the evidence. Doses vary widely among studies and among individuals, making comparison and generalization of findings difficult. Also, the interaction of substances with other factors, such as the environment, genetics, and preexisting mental health, can influence outcomes significantly.

Research in the field of microdoses has also faced legal and funding barriers. Legal restrictions around psychedelic substances have limited the amount and quality of research that can be conducted. Lack of funding and stigma associated with psychedelic substances have also hampered more extensive and larger studies.

Although there is emerging evidence that suggests possible benefits of microdoses in terms of cognitive improvement, creativity, and mental health, it is necessary to be critical in assessing the quality and reliability of this evidence. Stronger, well-designed, controlled studies are needed to draw firmer conclusions about the effects and benefits of microdoses. Until then, it is prudent to consider the available evidence as a starting point for future research and to guide informed and responsible decision-making regarding microdoses of psychedelic and ancestral substances.

IDENTIFICATION OF PROMISING AREAS AND LIMITATIONS IN CURRENT RESEARCH

Current research on microdoses of psychedelic and ancestral substances has identified promising areas and at the same time faces several limitations that deserve detailed analysis. In promising areas, it is encouraging to note the growing interest in exploring the potential effects and benefits of microdoses on mental health and general well-being. The focus on therapeutic potential and cognitive improvement has prompted research that could shed light on novel ways to address disorders such as anxiety, depression, and lack of concentration.

Initial studies have also revealed evidence that microdoses can have a positive impact on creativity and cognitive flexibility. This could have applications in fields such as art, music, and innovation, where the focus on enhancing creativity is of great value. In addition, the field of neuroscience has begun to explore how microdoses influence brain connectivity, which could help to better understand the underlying mechanisms of observed effects.

However, it is important to address the limitations that current research faces. First, the lack of placebo-controlled, double-blind studies is a significant obstacle. The absence of a control group and the difficulty of blind studies due to the nature of psychedelic substances limit the ability to attribute observed effects directly to microdoses. This raises questions about whether the results are a product of the actual effects of the substances or whether they are due to factors such as expectations and placebo effects.

Another limitation is the lack of standardization in terms of dosage and substances used in microdoses. The diversity in doses and types of substances makes it difficult to compare and generalize the results between different studies. In addition, interactions with other factors, such as pre-existing mental health and the environment, can influence outcomes and make it difficult to attribute effects exclusively to microdoses.

Legal restrictions are also a significant constraint on research. Stigma and regulations surrounding psychedelic substances have made it difficult to conduct robust, funded studies. This has led to a lack of funds and resources to conduct large-scale, well-controlled research that can provide a stronger understanding of the effects of microdoses.

In short, while current research on microdoses offers promising areas and reveals potential benefits in mental health and creativity, it is vital to recognize and address the inherent limitations. Experimental design, lack of standardization and legal restrictions present significant challenges in obtaining reliable and generalizable evidence. Overcoming these constraints will require greater investment in rigorous, well-designed research, together with a clear understanding of the ethical and legal frameworks within which research in this emerging field operates.

LIST OF SCIENTIFIC STUDIES ON THE USE OF SUBSTANCES

In a study by Carhart-Harris et al (2016), psilocybin, a component of magic mushrooms, was administered to patients with treatment-resistant depression. The results showed a significant reduction in symptoms of depression and an improvement in quality of life. However, this study did not specifically focus on microdoses.

Another exploratory study conducted by Schmid et al. (2018) analyzed the effects of LSD microdose on creativity. Participants reported increased creativity and open-mindedness, although the methodology had limitations in terms of the lack of control group.

In 2016, Griffiths and others examined the effects of psilocybin on cancer patients experiencing existential anxiety. Although this study did not focus on microdoses, a single dose of psilocybin was found to lead to sustained decreases in anxiety and depression over several months.

Following the literature of scientific studies, in one published by Fadiman and Korb (2019), anecdotal reports of people who performed LSD microdoses were collected. Participants reported improvements in concentration, creativity, and mood, although the results lacked a control group and no objective data was collected.

A pilot study led by Smigielski et al. (2019) explored the effects of psilocybin on mindfulness meditation. Participants reported greater depth in their meditation practices and greater connection with themselves and their environment.

These studies provide an initial view of the possible therapeutic and experiential effects of psychedelic substances, but it is important to note that most of them did not focus exclusively on microdoses and, for the most part, have methodological limitations and small samples. While these results are encouraging, more extensive and rigorous research is needed to fully understand the benefits and risks of microdoses in different contexts.

MICRODOSING AND MENTAL HEALTH

EXPLORING THE PATHS TO A MIND IN BALANCE

In the previous chapters, we have immersed our minds in the fundamentals, substances, and evidence base of microdoses. Now, we enter a territory of profound interest and relevance: the impact of microdoses on mental well-being. In this chapter, we will explore how these small doses of substances can play a role in promoting a healthier and more balanced mind.

Mental health is an essential component of our human experience. In a world that often challenges us with stress, anxiety, and other concerns, an intriguing question arises: can microdoses provide a path to relief and personal transformation? Throughout these pages, we will explore this question from multiple angles.

We will unravel how microdoses can influence the emotional and cognitive aspects of our lives. Can they contribute to reducing anxiety and depression? Is there evidence to support mood-boosting and creativity-boosting? Through a close look at scientific studies and subjective experiences, we will seek to understand the implications of microdoses on mental well-being.

However, we will also address the inherent complexities of this topic. We recognize that solutions are not always universal and that what works for one individual may not be right for another. Microdoses may be a powerful tool, but they are not a panacea. Therefore, we will discuss the importance of individualization, the multidimensional approach to mental health and how microdoses could be integrated into a broader plan of self-care.

As we explore the connections between microdoses and mental wellbeing, it is crucial to maintain a balanced, evidence-based approach. Stories of individuals who have experienced improvements in their mental health due to microdoses are valuable, but they must be contextualized within the broader scientific framework. By understanding both possibilities and limitations, we will be better prepared to make informed decisions about how to address our own mental health and explore pathways to a balanced mind.

EXPLORING HOW MICRODOSES CAN IMPACT MENTAL HEALTH

The relationship between microdoses and mental well-being has been a topic of growing interest in recent years. Although research in this area is still in its initial stages, there is anecdotal evidence and exploratory studies that suggest that microdoses of psychedelic substances could have a positive impact on mental health.

One of the most promising aspects is the possible influence of microdoses on mood disorders, such as depression and anxiety. Some anecdotal reports and preliminary studies have noted that people who performed microdoses experienced a decrease in depressive and anxiety symptoms. It has been speculated that psychedelic substances can modulate brain activity and emotional perception, which could contribute to these beneficial effects. However, it is important to note that this area still requires more robust and controlled research to establish clear conclusions.

In addition to mood disorders, microdoses may also influence other aspects of mental health, such as creativity and self-exploration. It has been observed in exploratory studies that microdoses can increase cognitive flexibility and mental openness, which could have implications in the generation of ideas and in artistic and scientific creativity. Also, some people have reported that microdoses have allowed them to explore aspects of themselves that are not normally accessible, which could have implications for self-acceptance and self-exploration.

However, it is essential to address the limitations of current research in this area. Most studies are small and lack adequate control groups. The variability in reported effects and the difficulty to perform double-blind studies due to the nature of psychedelic substances are significant challenges. In addition, the lack of standardization in terms of dosage and substances used in microdoses makes it difficult to compare results between different studies.

Microdoses of psychedelic substances have the potential to influence mental well-being, especially in areas such as depression, anxiety, creativity, and self-exploration.

While the current evidence is promising, it is important to consider methodological limitations and the need for more controlled and rigorous research. Understanding how microdoses can impact mental health is an evolving field that has the potential to offer new perspectives in treatment and improvement of emotional well-being.

POTENTIAL THERAPEUTIC APPLICATIONS IN DISORDERS SUCH AS ANXIETY, DEPRESSION, AND POST-TRAUMATIC STRESS

Potential therapeutic applications of microdoses in disorders such as anxiety, depression and post-traumatic stress disorder have generated great interest in the scientific and medical community. While research is in its preliminary stages, there are indications that microdoses of psychedelic substances could offer an innovative approach to addressing these mental health disorders.

In the case of anxiety, preliminary studies suggest that microdoses may have an anxiolytic effect. Some individuals who have taken microdoses have reported a decrease in anxiety levels and an increase in the sense of calm. It has been speculated that this could be due to modulation of brain circuits related to the response to stress and anxiety. However, it is crucial to stress that anxiety is a complex phenomenon and that more solid research is needed to determine the efficacy of microdoses as treatment.

In the case of depression, anecdotal reports and some exploratory studies suggest that microdoses could have a positive impact on improving mood.

Some participants in these studies have reported a reduction in depressive symptoms and an increase in motivation and vitality. However, controlled, large-scale studies are necessary to fully understand how microdoses might influence neurochemistry and brain connectivity associated with depression.

About post-traumatic stress disorder, there are indications that microdoses could play a role in managing symptoms. Some anecdotal reports suggest that microdoses could help people cope and process past trauma more effectively. It has been theorized that psychedelic substances could facilitate cognitive measurement and controlled exposure to traumatic memories, which could be beneficial for some individuals.

However, it is essential to emphasize that the therapeutic application of microdoses in these disorders is a complex and delicate area. The doses, frequency, and duration of microdoses should be carefully considered and personalized for each individual. In addition, possible adverse effects and associated risks need to be considered, especially in vulnerable populations.

Potential therapeutic applications of microdoses in disorders such as anxiety, depression, and post-traumatic stress disorder present fertile ground for research. While the results so far are encouraging, rigorous and controlled studies are needed to establish the efficacy and safety of microdoses as a complement or alternative to conventional therapeutic approaches. The focus on personalization and caution is essential when considering microdoses as part of the treatment strategy in mental health.

INTEGRATION OF MICRODOSES IN TRADITIONAL AND ALTERNATIVE MEDICINE

EXPLORING THE BRIDGE BETWEEN TRADITIONAL AND ALTERNATIVE MEDICINE

As we journey through the fundamentals of microdoses, we have unraveled their history, the substances that make them up, scientific research, and their relationship to mental wellbeing. Now, we move into an exciting field: integrating microdoses into the context of current medical practice. In this chapter, we will explore how these small doses can build a bridge between traditional and alternative medicine.

Medicine is a constantly evolving field, and the openness to unconventional approaches is more evident than ever. Microdoses represent a unique fusion of ancient wisdom and modern perspectives. In this chapter, we will examine how medical professionals and patients can navigate this fertile terrain in an informed and collaborative manner.

We will explore the ethical and legal implications of integrating microdoses into medical practice. How is the doctor-patient relationship managed when unconventional approaches are considered? What is the role of self-regulation and accountability in this area? As the medical community considers new perspectives, it is critical to maintain a transparent dialog and evidence-based approach.

We will also explore concrete examples of how microdoses could complement or integrate with other medical treatments. From anxiety disorders and depression to chronic pain management, we will examine where microdoses could offer added value and how such integrative approaches could be structured.

In addition, we will consider how medical professionals can receive training and education on microdoses. The intersection between traditional and alternative medicine often requires a change in mindset and the acquisition of new knowledge. We will therefore address the resources available and how physicians can be well equipped to make informed decisions for the benefit of their patients.

As we explore the integration of microdoses into medical practice, it is essential to maintain an open mind and collaborative spirit. Medicine is a diverse and constantly evolving field, and microdoses are just one example of how therapeutic approaches can adapt and expand. By building bridges between traditional and alternative medicine, we can contribute to a more patient-centered and comprehensive medical landscape that embraces both the science and the wisdom accumulated over the centuries.

HOW MEDICAL PROFESSIONALS CAN INCORPORATE MICRODOSES INTO THEIR THERAPEUTIC APPROACH

The incorporation of microdoses in the therapeutic approach of medical professionals is a topic that has generated a significant debate in the medical and mental health community. While there is a growing interest in exploring the possibilities of microdoses as an adjunct to conventional treatments, there are also ethical, legal, and scientific challenges that need to be carefully addressed.

First, it is essential that medical professionals become familiar with current scientific research on microdoses and psychedelic substances. This involves being aware of the latest studies, conclusions, protocols, and potential therapeutic applications. Continuous education and constant updating are essential to ensure that professionals have an informed and up-to-date knowledge.

In addition, informed decision-making is crucial when considering microdoses as part of the therapeutic approach. Practitioners should consider available evidence, weigh potential benefits and risks, and openly discuss these options with their patients. Open communication and transparency are essential to enable patients to make informed decisions and actively participate in their own treatment.

Interdisciplinary consultation is also recommended when considering microdoses. Working in partnership with psychologists, therapists, and other mental health professionals can enrich the patient's understanding and ensure a holistic approach to treatment. The experience in psychotherapy and the knowledge of emotional dynamics can be complementary to the integration of microdoses in the therapeutic process.

However, it is vital to stress that the incorporation of microdoses in medical practice poses ethical and legal challenges. Regulations around psychedelic substances vary by location and can have serious legal consequences. Practitioners should be aware of the legal and ethical implications and ensure that any therapeutic approach involving microdosing is consistent with local laws and regulations.

In summary, the incorporation of microdoses into the therapeutic approach of medical professionals requires a solid base of scientific knowledge, informed and ethical decision-making, and interdisciplinary collaboration. While microdoses show promising therapeutic potential, it is essential that practitioners follow the highest standards of medical care and ethics when considering this option. Continuous education and openness to dialog are essential to guide this evolution in medical practice.

ETHICAL AND LEGAL CONSIDERATIONS IN THE RECOMMENDATION OF MICRODOSES TO PATIENTS

Ethical and legal considerations in recommending microdoses to patients are essential for any health care practitioner considering this therapeutic approach. The controversial nature and legal regulation of psychedelic substances pose significant challenges that must be addressed with responsibility and caution.

From an ethical perspective, health professionals have the primary responsibility to prioritize the safety and well-being of their patients. When considering the recommendation for microdosing, they should carefully evaluate the available scientific evidence and consider whether the potential benefits outweigh the potential risks. The lack of comprehensive and controlled research in the field of microdoses implies considerable uncertainty in terms of effects and safety, which requires a cautious approach.

Patient autonomy must also be respected. Practitioners should provide complete and accurate information about microdoses, possible effects, and risks and allow patients to make informed decisions. Also, patients should be aware of the legal implications and potential impacts on their life, such as employment, relationships, and other areas.

As for legal considerations, regulations around psychedelic substances vary in different countries and jurisdictions. Some substances are completely banned, while others may be controlled or allowed only for medical and research purposes. Practitioners should be aware of local laws and regulations and ensure that any therapeutic approach involving microdoses is consistent with the law.

Recommending microdoses to patients also raises questions about the health care practitioner's professionalism and reputation. Given that microdoses are still an emerging and controversial field, some colleagues and society in general may question the integrity and motivations of the professional recommending them. It is critical that practitioners address these concerns openly and transparently, by providing research-supported information and by defending their ethical and evidence-based approach.

Ethical and legal considerations in the recommendation of microdoses to patients are fundamental to guarantee the safety, well-being, and rights of patients, as well as the professionalism of the health professional.

Evaluation of evidence, promotion of patient autonomy, and compliance with legal regulations are essential components of this process. In such a novel and controversial field, decision-making must be guided by strong ethical principles and a thorough understanding of the legal implications.

COLLABORATION BETWEEN TRADITIONAL MEDICINE AND ALTERNATIVE MEDICINE IN THE USE OF MICRODOSES

The collaboration between traditional medicine and alternative medicine in the use of microdoses is a topic that reflects the evolution and convergence of therapeutic approaches as our understanding of health and well-being broadens. As conventional and alternative medicine continue to explore new ways to address patients' needs, the integration of microdoses as a potential tool presents opportunities for dialog and synergy between the two fields.

Traditional medicine is based on practices and treatments that have been widely tested and supported by scientific evidence. However, the growing acceptance of complementary and alternative approaches has opened the door to the exploration of therapies that were previously considered marginal. Microdoses are at this crossroads, being considered an alternative and promising intervention that could complement or expand the available treatment options.

Collaboration between the two disciplines could bring unique perspectives. Traditional medicine can offer a rigorous evidence-based approach, while alternative medicine can provide a holistic, individual-centered understanding of health. By exploring microdoses, both disciplines could contribute to research and understanding of their therapeutic effects in a variety of conditions.

It is essential that this collaboration be based on transparency, mutual respect, and knowledge-sharing. Professionals in both disciplines should be open to learning and understanding the perspectives of the other field, as well as sharing their own experience and knowledge regarding microdoses. Interdisciplinarity in research and practice could allow for a more comprehensive and robust approach in assessing the benefits and risks of microdoses in therapeutic contexts.

However, it is important to recognize that the collaboration between traditional and alternative medicine in the use of microdoses also presents challenges. Differences in research methodology, legal regulation, and belief systems can generate conflicts and obstacles to effective collaboration. Moreover, the lack of a solid basis for controlled research in the field of microdoses requires a careful and ethical approach.

In continuing this collaboration between traditional and alternative medicine in the use of microdoses, it is essential to address key issues to ensure that patients receive safe and effective treatment. One of the crucial areas is the education and training of professionals in both disciplines. Clinicians and therapists should have a solid understanding of psychedelic substances, their possible effects, and risks, as well as interactions with other treatments and drugs.

Fluid communication between professionals is also essential to ensure comprehensive care. Patients exploring microdoses may be receiving alternative medical treatments or therapies, and it is essential that practitioners are aware of all interventions being used. This can help prevent negative interactions and create a consistent, personalized approach for the patient.

Data collection and joint research are also crucial aspects of this collaboration. Traditional medicine brings a rigorous scientific approach to research, while alternative medicine can contribute holistic perspectives and patient experiences. By working together on research projects, practitioners can help generate compelling evidence about the effects and benefits of microdoses in a variety of health conditions.

However, as collaboration progresses, it is important to address ethics and responsibility in relation to the promotion of microdoses. Misleading or exaggerated advertising can jeopardize patient trust and undermine the ethical foundations of medicine. It is essential that practitioners promote accurate, evidence-supported information and avoid creating unrealistic expectations in patients.

The collaboration between traditional and alternative medicine in the use of microdoses presents an exciting opportunity to explore innovative and holistic therapies. However, this collaboration must be based on education, communication, research, and ethics. By working together, practitioners can leverage their unique strengths to provide a comprehensive, personalized approach to the well-being of patients looking to explore microdoses as part of their treatment.

The collaboration between traditional medicine and alternative medicine in the use of microdoses is an opportunity to broaden the therapeutic approach and explore new frontiers in the treatment of various conditions. But this collaboration must be guided by ethics, transparency, and a willingness to learn and share knowledge. Interdisciplinarity in research and practice could allow a more comprehensive and evidence-based approach in the exploration of microdoses as a therapeutic tool.

THE FUTURE OF MICRODOSING

EXPLORING HORIZONS TO DISCOVER IN THE PRACTICE OF MICRODOSES

We have come a fascinating way through the fundamentals, substances, scientific evidence, mental well-being, and medical integration in the world of microdoses. Now, at the high point of our journey, we find ourselves at the crossroads of the future. In this chapter, we will explore the exciting possibilities and unknowns that lie ahead on the horizon of microdoses.

Interest in microdoses has grown exponentially in recent years, opening an interdisciplinary dialog that encompasses medicine, psychology, neuroscience, and culture in general. As we go through this exploration, we ask: what could be the role of microdoses in the future of health, well-being, and personal evolution?

In this chapter, we will reflect on emerging trends in scientific research and public acceptance of microdoses. What progress could we expect in terms of regulation and legitimization? How could microdoses help address mental and emotional health challenges in an increasingly complex world?

We will explore how microdoses might influence culture and society in the future. Could these practices change our perspective on medicine, mental health, and spirituality? How could they be integrated into educational and therapeutic contexts more broadly?

In addition, we will discuss the possible directions of scientific research in relation to microdoses. What questions still do not have clear answers? Where could we expect significant advances in understanding the mechanisms behind microdoses?

It is crucial to address both the possibilities and the limitations as we envision the future of microdoses. Despite their potential, these practices also raise ethical questions and practical challenges. In doing so, we will forge an informed and balanced perspective on what could come in the exciting and evolutionary field of microdoses.

PERSPECTIVES ON HOW THE FIELD OF MICRODOSES WILL EVOLVE IN THE COMING YEARS

Prospects for how the microdose field will evolve in the coming years are cautiously optimistic, driven by growing public and scientific interest in psychedelic substances and their potential therapeutic applications. As research continues to advance and new dialogs around mental health and wellbeing are opened, microdoses are expected to play an increasingly key role in medical care.

One of the main factors that will contribute to the evolution of the field is the expansion of scientific research. As more rigorous and controlled studies of microdoses are conducted, a deeper understanding of their effects, mechanisms of action, and potential therapeutic applications is expected. This stronger scientific evidence could support the integration of microdoses into conventional treatments and lead to regulatory approval in certain medical settings.

In addition, the evolution of the field will depend on the attitude of society and health systems towards psychedelic substances. As perceptions change and psychedelic substances are de-stigmatized, more medical professionals and therapists are likely to be willing to explore microdoses as part of a comprehensive therapeutic approach. However, addressing ethical, legal and safety concerns will also be essential to ensure that microdoses are used responsibly and effectively.

The collaboration between traditional medicine and alternative medicine could also have a significant impact on the evolution of the field. As different disciplines share their knowledge and perspectives, more comprehensive and personalized therapeutic approaches could emerge that leverage the best of both worlds. Interaction between practitioners in different areas can generate stronger research and guide how microdoses are applied in different clinical settings.

The evolution of the microdose field will also depend on government regulation and health policies. As clearer legal frameworks are established and more extensive research is allowed, opportunities for therapeutic application of microdoses are likely to expand. However, it is important to note that regulations can vary widely by country and jurisdiction, which could affect the availability and accessibility of microdoses in different locations.

The evolution of the microdose field will depend on the combination of scientific research, social acceptance, interdisciplinary collaboration, and regulatory developments. If ethical, legal, and scientific challenges are effectively addressed, microdoses may find a legitimate place in health care and wellbeing in the coming years. However, it is important to remember that the field is constantly evolving and that an informed and evidence-based approach will be needed to guide its development in a responsible and beneficial manner.

POTENTIAL FOR GREATER ACCEPTANCE AND REGULATION

The potential for greater acceptance and regulation of microdoses in the future is an issue that reflects the changing evolution of social, scientific, and political perspectives around psychedelic substances. As research continues to shed light on the potential therapeutic benefits of microdoses and challenges the historical stigma associated with these substances, it is plausible that we will see a gradual shift toward greater acceptance and more sensible regulation.

Public acceptance is undergoing a significant transformation as conversations about mental health, wellbeing, and alternative therapies become more open and broader. As stories are shared of people who have experienced significant benefits through microdosing, a more informed and empathetic dialog is being generated around these substances. The demand for more holistic and effective treatment options is driving the exploration of novel approaches, including microdoses.

Scientific research is playing a crucial role in generating evidence to support the potential efficacy of microdoses. As rigorous studies continue, a clearer understanding of the specific mechanisms of action, effects, and therapeutic applications of microdoses is likely to emerge. This evidence supported by science could be a determining factor in the evolution of acceptance and regulation.

In terms of regulation, some jurisdictions are already considering more pragmatic approaches to psychedelic substances. In some places, changes in drug policies are taking place that reflect a more nuanced understanding of the risks and benefits of these substances. Decriminalizing or legalizing certain psychedelic substances for medical or therapeutic purposes could pave the way for more regulated use of microdoses.

But it is important to note that regulation also presents challenges. The need to establish safe dosage standards, ensure product quality and prevent misuse are key considerations that need to be addressed in any regulatory framework. In addition, the education and training of medical professionals and therapists are essential to ensure that microdoses are used responsibly and effectively.

The potential for greater acceptance and regulation of microdoses will depend on a careful balance between scientific evidence, public acceptance, and government policies. As society becomes more informed and open, and as research progresses, we may see a shift in perception and focus around microdoses. However, this process will require a deliberate, collaborative approach that considers potential therapeutic benefits, safety, and ethical and legal implications.

POTENTIAL SCIENTIFIC AND THERAPEUTIC ADVANCES RELATED TO MICRODOSES

The possible scientific and therapeutic advances related to microdoses are a source of excitement and expectation in the scientific and medical community. As research on psychedelic substances and their therapeutic applications continues to advance, several areas are emerging where we could see considerable progress in the coming years.

One of the most anticipated advances concerns the understanding of the mechanisms of action of microdoses in the brain. Although much remains to be discovered, substances such as LSD and psilocybin have been shown to interact with neurotransmitter systems and brain networks that play a crucial role in regulating mood, perception, and cognition. As brain imaging technology and neural mapping techniques become more sophisticated, a more detailed understanding of how microdoses affect brain circuits and how this translates into potential therapeutic benefits is likely to be gained.

Another promising development relates to the identification of specific therapeutic applications. While there are indications that microdoses could be useful in treating disorders such as anxiety, depression and post-traumatic stress disorder, rigorous research is beginning to explore how microdoses could be applied more specifically in different clinical contexts. New areas in which microdoses can make a difference, such as managing chronic pain, enhancing creativity, or even promoting neuroplasticity, may be discovered.

Research could also reveal ways to optimize the doses, frequency, and duration of microdoses to obtain the best therapeutic results. Determining "effective microdosing" is a key challenge, and progress in customizing interventions based on individual characteristics could be a major trend. This could include identifying biomarkers that help predict an individual's response to microdoses and adjusting doses accordingly.

In addition, research around microdoses could lead to a greater understanding of brain plasticity and the reconfiguration of thinking and behavior patterns. This could have therapeutic implications not only for specific disorders, but also for promoting general well-being and personal growth.

The potential scientific and therapeutic advances associated with microdoses are numerous and exciting. As research continues to advance and public acceptance evolves, we may be on the verge of discoveries that transform the way we approach mental health and wellbeing. However, these advances will require a rigorous, collaborative, and ethical approach to ensure that microdoses are used safely, effectively, and responsibly in the context of health care and therapy.

CONCLUSION

In this book, we have explored a broad spectrum of knowledge related to microdoses and their potential impact on mental health and well-being. From its foundations to its therapeutic applications, from its relationship with traditional medicine to its future evolution, we have traveled a journey that has led us to understand the complexities and promises surrounding this emerging approach.

We began with a solid foundation, laying the foundations of microdoses and their historical evolution. From the ancestral use of plants and psychedelic substances in spiritual ceremonies to their resurgence in contemporary research, we have observed how microdoses have been a constant in various cultures and eras. This historical understanding is essential to contextualize the current emergence of microdoses as a possible therapeutic tool.

We explore in depth how microdoses interact with the body and mind, revealing their mechanisms of action and their possible beneficial effects. We learned that microdoses can modulate neurotransmitter systems and brain networks, impacting areas related to cognition, perception, and emotions. This understanding allowed us to glimpse how microdoses could have therapeutic applications, especially in the field of mental well-being.

In our analysis of the non-psychedelic and psychedelic substances used in microdoses, we discovered a variety of compounds ranging from ancestral plants to synthetic substances. Each of these substances offers potential mental health benefits, from improving focus and reducing stress to expanding awareness and promoting creativity. However, we recognized the importance of research and prudence in considering its use.

The integration of microdoses into medical and therapeutic practice was another key issue that we addressed. We consider how medical professionals can incorporate microdoses ethically and effectively in their therapeutic approach, collaborating with traditional and alternative medicine to provide comprehensive and personalized care. We also explore ethical and legal considerations in recommending microdoses to patients, stressing the importance of safety, transparency, and informed decision-making.

Scientific research and empirical evidence occupied a principal place in our exploration. We examined studies investigating the effects of microdoses on various mental health conditions, which shed light on their therapeutic potential. We also critically evaluate the quality and reliability of available evidence, identifying promising areas and limitations in current research.

We consider how microdoses can impact mental well-being and explore possible therapeutic applications in disorders such as anxiety, depression, and post-traumatic stress. We recognized that while the potential is encouraging, more research is needed to fully understand its benefits and risks in different clinical settings.

Finally, we reflect on the future of microdoses and their evolution in the coming years. We see increasing acceptance and regulation, driven by ever-advancing scientific research and the evolution of social attitudes towards psychedelic substances. We consider the possible scientific and therapeutic advances that could arise, from a deeper understanding of the mechanisms of action to the identification of more specific and personalized therapeutic applications.

Together, this book has been a journey of exploration and understanding of microdoses and their potential to improve mental well-being. While we have addressed many key aspects, it is important to recognize that the field of microdoses remains dynamic and evolving. The path to a comprehensive understanding and effective therapeutic use of microdoses requires an informed, ethical, and evidence-based approach, guided by a commitment to improving people's mental health and wellbeing.

Susan McDowell

A FINAL WORD

At a time when mental health and wellbeing are more important than ever, we have a unique opportunity to drive forward research in a promising and still under-explored area: the therapeutic potential of psychedelic substances and microdoses. While we have come a long way in understanding these substances, there is still vast territory to explore and discover. That is why we call on the medical community and the public to unite in the search for more visibility and funding in studies with psychedelic substances.

The potential benefits of psychedelic substances in mental health have begun to emerge, supported by a growing scientific evidence base. However, to fully exploit its therapeutic potential, it is imperative that we promote greater investment in research. We need robust and rigorous studies exploring the mechanisms of action, clinical applications, and safety of these substances. An investment in research will not only broaden our understanding, but could also open the door to revolutionary treatments for conditions like depression, anxiety, and post-traumatic stress disorder.

To achieve this goal, we urge the medical community to join in the drive towards greater visibility and funding in studies with psychedelic substances. Health professionals have the power to bring about meaningful change by supporting and actively participating in rigorous and ethical research in this field. In addition, it is essential that they share their knowledge and experiences with colleagues and patients, thereby contributing to an informed and evidence-based conversation about the therapeutic potential of psychedelic substances.

At the same time, we call on the public to join this cause. We are all involved in promoting the mental health and well-being of our communities. By supporting research organizations, raising awareness, and promoting open and respectful conversations, we can raise the visibility of psychedelic research and foster an enabling environment for the necessary funding.

To cultivate genuine self-control, it is essential to distinguish between the true rewards that imbue our lives with meaning and the deceptive rewards that merely serve to distract and entrap us in cycles of addiction. True rewards are those that align with our core values and contribute to our long-term well-being. They include fulfilling relationships, personal growth, and achievements that resonate deeply with our sense of purpose. Engaging with these rewards requires effort, patience, and a commitment to our overarching life goals. They provide a lasting sense of satisfaction and enrich our lives in meaningful ways, reinforcing our intrinsic motivations and leading to sustainable happiness.

In contrast, false rewards are often immediate and superficial, designed to captivate our attention and provide short-lived pleasure. These can manifest as excessive screen time, compulsive shopping, unhealthy eating habits, or substance abuse. While they may offer temporary gratification, they leave us feeling empty and craving more, creating a vicious cycle of dependency. To break free from this cycle, we must become mindful of the difference between what truly nourishes our spirit and what merely distracts us. By consciously choosing activities and goals that offer real, substantial rewards, we can foster self-discipline and create a more fulfilling, purpose-driven life.

Microdosing is about self-control and exploration of experiences that could have a deep impact in your life.

Research on psychedelic substances has the potential to revolutionize mental health treatment. But to get to that point, we must join in a collective effort to increase visibility and funding in studies in this field. The medical community and the public have a vital role to play in this process. Together, we can drive research, de-stigmatize these substances, and work toward a future in which treatment options are broader, more effective, and more hopeful for all.

RESOURCES

Websites:

PubMed - https://pubmed.ncbi.nlm.nih.gov/
Medscape - https://www.medscape.com/
WebMD - https://www.webmd.com/
Mayo Clinic - https://www.mayoclinic.org/
CDC (Centers for Disease Control and Prevention) - https://www.cdc.gov/

Books:

"Harrison's Principles of Internal Medicine" - Author: Dennis Kasper, Anthony Fauci, et al.
"Gray's Anatomy for Students" - Author: Richard Drake, Wayne Vogl, et al.
"The Merck Manual of Diagnosis and Therapy" - Editor: Robert S. Porter.
"Robbins and Cotran Pathologic Basis of Disease" - Author: Vinay Kumar, Abul K. Abbas, et al.
"Current Medical Diagnosis and Treatment" - Author: Maxine Papadakis, Stephen McPhee, et al.

Studies:

Study on Psilocybin for Treatment-Resistant Depression, Carhart-Harris et al. (2016).
Microdose Research by LSD and Creativity, Schmid et al. (2018).
Study on Psilocybin and Existential Anxiety, Griffiths et al. (2016).
LSD Microdose and Cognition Research, Fadiman and Korb (2019).
Study on Psilocybin and Mindfulness, Smigielski et al. (2019).

ABOUT SUSAN MCDOWELL

In the dynamic world of health and wellness, Dr. Susan McDowell stands out as a visionary and a beacon of knowledge, profoundly dedicated to empowering individuals to reach their full potential. Her journey in medicine is not merely a career, but a lifelong pursuit of understanding and sharing the intricacies of human well-being.

Dr. McDowell's foundational expertise was forged at the prestigious University of Medicine and Health Sciences, where she earned her medical degree. This rigorous academic background laid the groundwork for a professional path characterized by a unique blend of hands-on clinical expertise and an unwavering commitment to research. For years, she has cultivated her own medical practice, earning not only the respect but also the deep admiration of her patients through her compassionate care.

Beyond the clinic, Susan McDowell has forged an innovative path as a prolific writer, extending her influence far beyond individual consultations. Her extensive writings are a testament to her profound medical knowledge, yet they offer something more: they distill her innate compassion and unwavering dedication to continuously improving the health and well-being of all who seek her guidance. Her publications resonate deeply, reflecting an integrative approach that has made meaningful contributions to the field. While the sources don't specify all her topics, the mention of "Going barefoot" alongside her medical background hints at the breadth and diverse nature of her explorations within health and wellness, reflecting her prolific output.

Through both her clinical practice and her impactful written works, Susan McDowell has firmly established herself as a highly respected figure in the expansive field of health and medicine, a testament to her holistic vision and relentless dedication. She truly embodies the spirit of a leading medical professional, constantly pushing the boundaries of knowledge for the betterment of others.

Beyond her impressive credentials and extensive knowledge, Dr. Susan McDowell's approach to healthcare is deeply rooted in her profound empathy and a genuinely warm, welcoming demeanor. Her clinical practice is more than just a place for medical consultation; it is a space where her deep passion for helping people reach their full potential truly shines through. This innate drive translates into an environment where patients feel not just treated, but genuinely understood and cared for.

Dr. McDowell's personal philosophy distills her compassion and unwavering commitment to the continuous improvement of the health and well-being of those who seek her guidance. It is this patient-centered approach, marked by a welcoming spirit and an admirable dedication, that has earned her not just the respect, but the deep admiration of her patients over many years in her own practice. While the sources primarily highlight her interactions with patients and those who seek her guidance, her demonstrated compassion and dedication suggest an intrinsically warm and supportive professional persona.

OTHER BOOKS BY THE AUTHOR

"Andropause Exposed: The Hidden Male Menopause, Low Testosterone, and the Secret to Reclaiming Energy, Strength, and Confidence"

The groundbreaking book, "Andropause Exposed: The Hidden Male Menopause, Low Testosterone, and the Secret to Reclaiming Energy, Strength, and Confidence," offers a comprehensive, empathetic, and empowering guide to understanding, managing, and thriving through these changes.

"Parenting without fear: A Guide to Loving Your Children"

Are you tired of parenting approaches rooted in anxiety, control, or endless struggles? For generations, many parenting practices have been influenced by underlying fears: fear of children not learning, not behaving, or not succeeding. These methods, often relying on pressures, rewards, or anger, can be not only ineffective but also deeply detrimental to a child's intrinsic drive for self-development. In 'Parenting without Fear,' we invite you to embark on a revolutionary journey that challenges conventional wisdom and reconsiders the very foundation of how you guide your children.

"Going barefoot: natural running, walking and movement to respect your body"

In "Going Barefoot: Natural Running, Walking and Movement to Respect Your Body," Susan McDowell delves into the profound benefits of reconnecting with the earth through natural movement. This insightful book emphasizes the importance of barefoot activities in fostering alignment, strength, and overall well-being. Drawing from both scientific research and her rich clinical experience, Susan offers practical advice and exercises to help readers embrace a more natural way of moving.

"Understanding SIBO: The Enigma of Small Intestinal Bacterial Overgrowth".

This book, the result of Susan's clinical experience, offers a clear and practical perspective on Small Intestinal Bacterial Overgrowth Syndrome (SIBO). Through her work, Susan unravels the mysteries of this condition, providing readers with an essential guide to understanding, addressing, and overcoming SIBO.

"Understanding Perimenopause: A Woman in Plenitude"

Discover the beauty in every change, from hormonal aspects to symptoms and body changes. With personal stories and anecdotes that resonate, you will feel accompanied in this unique chapter of your life. It explores how sexual health, emotional and psychological aspects, and general well-being intertwine in a journey full of authenticity and self-acceptance.

"Complete Guide to Red Light Therapy: Optimal Health, Healthy Skin and Other Benefits of Red Light."

As an advocate of holistic approaches to health, Susan explores the diverse benefits of red-light therapy in this book. From improving skin health to optimizing overall wellness, Susan's comprehensive guide offers valuable information backed by research, allowing readers to effectively integrate red light into their daily routine.

"Microdosing: Macrobenefits in health and well-being. Your body in psychedelic and non-psychedelic substances."

In her most innovative work, Susan explores the fascinating world of microdosing and its impacts on health and wellness. This book provides a balanced and scientifically grounded view on the use of psychedelic and non-psychedelic substances in microdosing, offering a unique perspective on their potential benefit to mental and emotional health.

"High-Need Babies, The Untold Truth: The Ultimate Parenting Guide for High-Demanding Childs (English Edition)"

Susan McDowell embarks on the journey of parenting with her English-language play "High-Need Babies." This book provides a unique and comprehensive insight for parents facing the challenge of raising children with high demands. With empathy and wisdom, Susan guides parents through effective strategies and offers an enlightening perspective on the particular needs of these children.

www.ingramcontent.com/pod-product-compliance
Lightning Source LLC
Chambersburg PA
CBHW061244250726
48653CB00002B/510